FULL THROTTLE... NO BREAKS

My life as a biker with ADHD

DUANE FERRIS

ISBN: 9781719912228

THANKYOU

A huge thanks goes to my long suffering wife
Shirley.
She has shown me love and understanding beyond
that which I deserve.
Love you forever xxx.

Big thanks to my friends and works colleagues,
Mark Williams, Janet Gillam and Steve Robinson
For bullying me into putting my words in print.
Love and respect to you all.

Finally, to my club brothers and sisters.
Always there for me as I am for you.

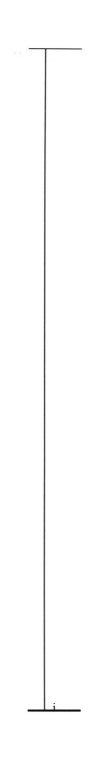

INTRODUCTION

No, the title is not a spelling mistake.

Attention Deficit Hyperactivity Disorder.
Attention Deficit Disorder.
Attention deficit hyperactivity disorder (ADHD) is a behavioural disorder that includes symptoms such as inattentiveness, hyperactivity and impulsiveness. Symptoms of ADHD tend to be noticed at an early age and may become more noticeable when a child's circumstances change, such as when they start school.
Or not.

I consider myself to be a biker and often wonder what started me down this path.
On a visit to my GP, she suggested that perhaps I would like to write about my experience of living with ADHD and a brain that has a broken pause button.

I was 54 years old before I even knew I had been living with this condition since birth.
It was only due to the job I do becoming increasingly less busy to a point of , more or less, doing nothing that I began to realise that something wasn't quite right and sought help.

My hope is that these words will help those with ADHD/ADD understand what's happening to them and for the people they share their lives with to have a little more understanding too.
There are many people who will claim that "There is no such thing as ADHD... there are just disruptive, naughty little brats !" I can assure you that there most certainly is such a thing and I'm all the proof I need.

I want to show that it's not all bad. In fact it can be very interesting if you let it. When I was a youngster it didn't even have a name and therefore did not exist. Only when you give something a name and let it control you does it become a problem. It was normal to me then, so why can't it be normal now?

I have tried to write this book in a similar way to which my mind works. At times it may seem a little

disjointed and suddenly fly off at a tangent but that's how I go through life.
I have written it in small sections because, if you have an attention span anything like mine, you would soon lose interest.

This book is about the way I see the World, that I am very much part of. If it offends anyone I can assure you that it was never my intention to do so. However, if you are offended, I think you'll find that the problem lies within yourself, not me.

I am not looking for sympathy or pity because none of this merits any, but If the following words can make just a single being feel better about themselves and not feel alone, it would all have been worthwhile.

What follows are my personal experiences and observations but I'm pretty sure you'll find something in there that you will recognise, even if you don't have this condition.

It has made me who I am today.... for better or worse.

CHAPTER 1

SOME NAMES HAVE BEEN CHANGED TO
PROTECT THE CULPABLE

*'I prefer to distinguish ADD as attention abundance
disorder. Everything is just so interesting . . .
remarkably at the same time.'*
*— **Frank Coppola, MA, ODC, ACG***

LYDBURY NORTH, SHROPSHIRE, SUMMER OF
1983

The distant, high pitched, metallic drone, of a two
stroke engine heralded the approach of an
unknown motorcycle. The sound was like a wasp,
wearing a suit of armour, trapped in a tin can and
getting rather annoyed.
Then it appeared, still a distant figure with a trail of
thin blue smoke from it's tail, screaming through the
sunny Shropshire countryside. It sliced through the
peaceful rural scene, sending birds back to the sky
and furry little rodents, that had ventured forth into

such a summer's day, quickly back to the safety of
the hedgerows.
A yellow and black Yamaha RD250 slid to a stop
beside us and the rider dismounted. The bike stood
there, balancing on it's own, like a cartoon
character that just realised it had gone past the
edge of a cliff, then fell with a clatter onto the
gravel. It's owner, wearing a battered, white open
face helmet and welding goggles, said nothing, just
reached into his pocket, pulled out a small
container, sprinkled a line of cocaine onto the side
of his hand, inhaled it all, waved, picked up the still
running bike and rode off in the direction of
wherever he happened to be pointing.
Perhaps this sounds a little odd ?.... not in my
World.
You meet all the best people on a motorcycle.

My overactive, unfocused mind was (and still is)
always looking for some sort of stimulation and,
despite my quiet nature, this often came along in
the form of something dangerous to my health and
thoroughly inadvisable. Although this rarely stopped
me from going ahead with it regardless.

When I was 16, I started work at a local frozen food
warehouse. Only a small operation that delivered to
local pubs and restaurants. When left to my own

devices I would climb the mountains of frozen chips boxes, walk tightropes of metal across the pallet frames and speed around, wheel Spinning the electric forklift truck. Somehow I remained unharmed and un-fired. The best part about the job is that I never got ill. Working at minus 20 degrees tends to kill off any germs that might want to have their evil way with your immune system.

One of the drivers was a strange fellow named Tecwyn. He was one of those people that could have been any age between 25 and 100 years old, it was impossible to tell. He spoke only in single syllables, usually "Ah", which was an answer to anything, positive or negative, depending on exactly how it was uttered and backed up with body language. His eyes pointed in completely different directions, which was a little disturbing when trying to communicate with him, especially when he always looked (and often smelled) like he had just crawled out of a rubbish skip. Despite his demeanour, he managed to get to work on a motorcycle... well, maybe not quite a motorcycle.

The Honda Express Scooter; 50 cubic centimetres of raw power. It was basically a pushbike with an engine bolted to it. No gears and a little shopping basket attached to the front. Yet because, for whatever reason I cannot recall, Tecwyn let me ride it around the car park. I was hooked.

I knew from that moment, as I barely missed colliding with the company fuel pump, that I had to have my own motorcycle.

A few days later, another driver, called Ken, took me for a ride on the back of his Honda 250 Superdream; a totally unremarkable motorcycle, but to me it was a monstrously powerful beast. Dangerous, exciting and totally cool.

I wanted one and I wanted it *right now*.

I soon found myself salivating over some nice shiny Kawasakis at a dealers in the centre of Chester. It was a bike dealers known as Newgate Motorcycles, that closed down at some point during the 1980s along with so many others.

What seemed at first to be a huge machine caught my eye. It was a bright green Kawasaki 125cc trials bike. I had gone there with no idea what I really wanted and had told my parents that I was looking for a moped, but there it was, a shiny new 'proper' motorcycle. Smiling at me and batting it's eyelashes.

Before I knew it, I had signed a finance contract, which included a cheap and nasty, polycarbonate, 'Centurian' helmet (which would later save my life), a pair of leather gauntlets and insurance.

It was only after I excitedly went to collect said machine that I realised I didn't have the slightest clue how to ride it. I had never used a clutch and gears before, let alone ridden anything with an engine attached. I started pushing it the 3 miles home, following numerous failed attempts at operating the beast that resulted in nothing but embarrassment.

On the route home I had to cross a large area of waste land, later to become a wasteland of cheap housing. I was rapidly losing the will to live and getting very tired, so attempted to ride the little green monster again. I simply couldn't get the knack of the clutch and was about to give up completely . After several more failures, a young lad of about 13 years appeared out of nowhere and said that if I let him have a go he would teach me how to ride. I agreed and soon enough got the hang of the whole clutch, throttle, brake thing and started making progress of sorts. At least I didn't need to push it any further.

My initial joy was a little deflated by the rather negative response of my parents; "What the hell have you bought that for?", "How can you afford that?","I thought you said you were buying a moped.", "You'll get yourself killed riding that!". The last bit was nearly true.

I spent the next few weeks falling in love with my new freedom. I fell off a couple of times on sheet ice and pulled a spectacular wheelie across the Chester Zoo traffic lights, entirely by accident. I imagine it looked rather spectacular, but it nearly needed a change of underwear on my part. Unfortunately, nobody had explained to me that the bike was a two stroke powered machine (not that I had any idea what that meant) and that I had to fill a small tank of two stroke oil, as well as putting petrol in the main tank. When the small tank ran out the bike stopped, rather suddenly.

Ah well, lesson learned, wallet much lighter, and the new found knowledge of what a rebore is.

The bike later repaid my ignorance by seizing the back brake, in torrential rain, during my driving test. Despite these lessons, I happily used the little Kawasaki to travel the 50 miles from Chester to RAF Cosford, where I was being trained to fix planes, in theory at least. It was a beautiful road at the time, with about a quarter of today's traffic. It slices through the Shropshire countryside, with lots of bendy bits and a few nice straight sections for overtaking.

The best thing about where I was stationed, to complete my trade training, was that it was full of bikers. Lots of 'em.

There is a big difference between a motorcyclist
and a biker, a huge difference in fact.
Anyone can buy a motorcycle and pass their test,
but that doesn't mean a thing to me, or anyone else
in my close circle of brothers from another mother.
What set my life on a different course was a single
gesture from a complete stranger.
I was riding into my home town of Chester, when I
saw another bike coming towards me. As we got
closer I realised that it was, what I regarded as, a
proper biker. He was riding an old British bike, loud
and dirty. He had an open face helmet with aviator
goggles perched on the brim and a black leather
jacket with a denim waistcoat over the top. A bright
smile was gleaming amongst all his facial hair, but
he still looked mean and raised an arm to
acknowledge me. *Me !...* this pale, scrawny kid on a
125cc bike, tootling along into town. I wobbled a
little and waved back.
From that moment on I wanted to be that guy. He
could have been a serial killer with a penchant for
wearing ladies underwear for all I knew, but I didn't
care. In that single moment I had been accepted
into a world that I would never look back from. I
was still a bit of a dork on a stupid green bike, but I
no longer cared.

If only I had known what lay ahead, I probably would have done it anyway.

I decided that the best course of action was to buy a black leather jacket, so I went ahead and bought one with long leather tassels on the back and arms. The shopping list also included black leather boots with white, knee length, wool socks that could be turned over the top of said boots. It also seemed appropriate to purchase a white silk scarf (it was in the rules).

There were no high tech items of clothing for bikers back then. If it rained you had fisherman's rubberized leggings or Belstaff,waxed cotton gear. If it was cold, you would don a wool 'donkey' jacket over your leather, wear silk glove liners and a thin balaclava. Basically you'd get wet and cold.

Helmets were not much better, they were noisy, poorly fitting and draughty. Visors would steam up within seconds and get covered in thousands of tiny scratches, so that oncoming headlight beams became refracted into a thousand points of light, rendering the rider blind for a few seconds. It was better to ride with the visor up most of the time, especially when it was raining and yes it hurt. Riding at speed in the rain is like having thousands of pins fired into your face. I won't even mention hailstones.

By now you're probably asking yourself, "What the hell has all of this got to do with ADHD?".
I shall explain…

Although, at the time, I had absolutely no idea what was going on in my head. I was an overly impulsive and easily influenced young idiot.
If something managed to catch my attention it would explode into hundreds of thoughts, visions and ideas.
When I decided to go down the route of becoming a biker, I wanted it to happen right there and then. I had little or no patience for anyone or anything that tried to stop me, but there was one huge barrier, parents.
They hated the whole idea of 2 wheels. It represented everything they were afraid of and betrayed every possible ideal they held dear for how their son should be seen.
In my mind this was brilliant, all the more reason to go ahead.
I started reading magazines like 'Easyrider' and 'Bike'. I got more and more into the rock music, that I already loved and became more and more detached from their vision of a perfect young man.
I must admit however, that at one point I even considered going down the scooter and Mod route.

My musical tastes are extremely varied and I still love SKA. Just not enough power, in both the machines and music.

The risk aspect of riding focused my wandering mind and because of the rapidly firing synapses, helped keep me alive.

There is an incredible amount of information bombarding the senses when you're on the road. I soon discovered that the best way to stay safe was to develop a belief that everyone else on the road were trying to kill me and couldn't even see me. Unfortunately both of these beliefs are quite often true.

The impulsiveness bit of ADHD, partly explains that, during my 36 years of riding, I have owned approximately 50 motorcycles, of various styles, ranging from old British thumpers to road legal race machines. Despite this fact, I hold a totally clean license (up to the point of writing this) and, although being involved in a couple of accidents, have never crashed a bike through loss of control or excess speed (and I have gone very fast indeed).

One of my biggest issues with ADHD and motorcycling is the imagining of every different possible scenario, any time I decide to go for a ride. This has often stopped me from going out at all.

Once I'm riding everything is fine, but leading up to the trip my stomach starts churning and I become restless, fidgety and impatient. I get snappy and agitated, just wanting to get on with it before I change my mind.

On the plus side I am rarely taken unawares by incidents on the road. I have literally been there, done that and bought the t-shirt, if only in my mind. Unfortunately it was one of those aforementioned drivers that either didn't see me or was actually trying to kill me that would change my life forever.

Fast forward to RAF Cosford, 1981…

There we were, the boys in blue, training to become flight systems technicians, without a care in the world, apart from me.

The lad who thought he'd escaped algebra when leaving school, soon discovered that he would be thrown head first into the deep end of algebraic equations on my first day of trade training. I was doomed.

Despite this I had a great time. I instantly made friends with whoever had a bike or liked rock music. There was my best mate, 'Wilco'. A punk come mod, with a very old Yamaha RD200, a history of drug abuse and a speech impediment. I distinctly remember the RAF Police investigation department coming to question him because he had an anti war poster on his wall along with one of Kate Bush injecting herself in the head. No sense of humour those guys.

Alan, on the other hand, was as straight as they came. Hated drugs and anything illegal, with a boring Honda 250 RS to match. He was alright I suppose, just lacking any sense of adventure or mischief. We swapped bikes one weekend and I wanted to give his back after 30 minutes. Far too sensible.

A crazy Scottish guy, who rarely spoke, known as 'Jock', for some reason, was part of our band of nutters. He owned a Yamaha RD350LC; a ridiculously fast 2 stroke machine that he would often just fall off, for no apparent reason, while going very fast in a straight line?

He managed this feat twice within a couple of weeks. He could provide us with no reason or explanation and we probably wouldn't have understood him anyway.

Anyone on camp with a bike of 500cc or over was considered to be a God. Such a person was Dave with his Ducati 860 GTS (in retrospect he was a complete dick head but we were young and easily impressed). It was a big, black and gold, v-twin, that sounded amazing and was relatively fast. It was just a shame about the rider.

The only exception to the 'God' rule was Tony and his old Triumph 650 Thunderbird. He spray can painted it in various shades of any colour available and the poor thing spent most of it's time in bits. He was basically insane, but a great laugh regardless. He was still a God I suppose, just a slightly demented one.

The main car park of the base was full of bikes, but our crew were much better, obviously.

One group decided that they would start a club called the 'Centurians MC' and had full back patches made with top and bottom rockers in red and white. I clearly remember the Wolverhampton chapter of the Hells Angels MC arriving at the camp gate, wanting to have a little chat with them, friendly like. They were, eventually, turned away at gunpoint by the lads on guard. However, the 'Centurians MC', miraculously, were never seen again. Lesson learned chaps. You can't just decide to become an MC club overnight, not without getting yourselves seriously hurt, or worse.

I was a bit of an anomaly back then, a biker with a skinhead that was also a bit of a hippy. I suppose I've always tried to be just that little bit different from the expected.

On that note I decided to spend what was a small fortune, in 1981 terms, on a Lewis Leathers jacket, not unusual except that it was bright red.

Made out of thick cowhide it could probably stop a bullet and because of it's excellent quality and strength I still have a right arm, but more of that later. On top of this jacket I wore the standard attire of a denim waistcoat adorned with a plethora of motorcycle badges and rock band patches. I had meticulously embroidered two band logos on the back (Van Halen and Rush) and the shoulders were covered in conical metal studs. I thought it was cool anyway. I wore an old, ragged and patched, pair of jeans over a newer pair and an embroidered cheesecloth kurta underneath my leather.

When not riding, I would wear flared jeans, a rust coloured 'Beatles' style jacket with weird, brass dangly bits on it and a corduroy waistcoat. The only thing missing was the long hair.

What was really missing was a bigger bike.

After the green machine spat out it's dummy during my bike test, in sunny Wolverhampton, by locking up the rear brake, I had to give up on the idea of buying a Triumph Bonneville, which was a blessing in disguise, and found a nice and very shiny Suzuki 250t. It was a laid back, custom cruiser, type of

thing that seemed huge to my fledgling biker brain.
I signed the finance agreement and a week later
got a lift from my fellow aircaftsman called Geordie,
for obvious reasons, in his Ford Granada, to collect
it.
I will never forget the feeling of riding that bike back
to the base. It was a sunny, late spring day and I
felt like the king of the world.
The Suzuki was smooth and powerful, comfortable
and cool. At least I thought it was. I felt like a
'proper' biker at last.
I spent every spare moment I had riding that bike
and I loved it. I relished the trip home along the A41
and rode like a madman, overtaking everything I
could and never dropping much below 80 mph.
How I didn't end up dead or seriously hurt still
escapes me.

I mentioned earlier about the poor quality of 80's
visors.
It was common practice to flip open your visor
when approaching roundabouts, or anything else
that needed unimpeded vision to negotiate safely.
This need occured whilst rapidly screaming towards
the Whitchurch truck stop roundabout, on my way
home from base.
I flicked open my visor, just as a very large bumble
bee was merrily and suicidedly flying towards my

face. It flew straight into my eye! I managed to keep control and clear my vision just as it's cousin chose exactly the same route, into exactly the same eye. I was lucky to survive this episode unharmed, but my eyes were streaming and it was a while before I was able to carry on my journey.

I don't know what it is about flying insects but they do seem rather intent on becoming multi coloured streaks on helmet visors.

Yes, they hurt and no, they don't taste very nice.

I was seriously into rock music by now. It suited my racing mind. The faster and louder the better. I would ride the bike to concerts anywhere and everywhere.

One such concert was taking place at Port Vale Football Club's ground, in Stoke on Trent. This event still holds the record for being one of the loudest open air concerts of all time. The headline band was Motorhead.... enough said.

The place was absolutely packed, the sun was shining and the promoters had sent everyone from the nearby elderly persons home on a day out to the seaside. There were a number of stalls selling small bottles of fizzy pop, which was fine until the temperature started rising and they followed suit by raising their prices. This resulted in a minor riot which included the stalls being ransacked and hundreds of plastic bottles being thrown into the stands, creating a fizzy, sticky and colourful waterfall of cheap pop cascading down the concrete steps. The vendors made a run for it.

The concert was excellent and I had the honour of seeing Ozzy Osbourne performing with the legendary guitarist Randy Rhoads, just before he died in a flying accident. A sad loss of an amazing talent.

When it was time to leave I discovered that Stoke is impossible to escape from. I got well and truly lost but soon found the M6 motorway. Off came the 'L' plates and I managed to find my way out towards Wolverhampton. It was a great buzz doing something I shouldn't and against the law. It felt rebellious, exciting and downright naughty. I got quite a buzz from that.

Forces living, once past the initial training, is quite a cosseted and easy life, if you don't mind being woken up at 3am, given a rifle and put on a 30mph restricted bus for a 200 mile trip up the M6, for a defensive exercise in Carlisle, now and then.

This left far too much time for my mind to become unoccupied and lacking in stimulation. My brain was buzzing away faster and faster, full of ideas and plans for the bike.

My trade training was getting me down. I could do absolutely anything practical that was put in front of me with ease. I could repair and build electrical equipment and was an expert on aerodynamics, but the dreaded algebra was holding me back. No matter how hard I tried to understand it, my brain just refused to make sense of it all, instantly dismissing it as unimportant and useless. The reality is that I have yet to find a single aircraft technician, mechanic or anyone involved in the general running of an aeroplane that has ever found the need to sit down and use algebra. I seriously doubt they ever will.

I was 'backflighted' after failing a maths (algebra) exam, which meant being put with a later class to try and catch up. I was away from all my mates and thinking to myself how little use this was going to be when I still couldn't do the maths, with little hope of that ever changing.

When an overactive mind gets depressed and bored stupid things begin to happen. I decided to take my perfectly decent looking Suzuki and strip all the paint off. Then I hand painted a very intricate design of swirling lines and mythical creatures on the tank and side panels. Being of a creative nature, it turned out rather well. It also turns out that I was wasting my time.

We all got sent home on 2 weeks leave in August 1981. I had started to spend more and more weekends staying on base with my buddies, so this was not a welcome break . I had booked a ticket for the 'Monsters of Rock' festival, being held at the Donnington race circuit in Derbyshire, during my time away from camp, in an attempt to break the boredom and quietude of home.

AC/DC were headlining, with their 'Back in Black' comeback tour, following the premature demise of their previous vocalist Bon Scott. After being bored silly at home for a week, I was really looking forward to something different.

On arrival I was met by grey skies, a muddy field and a bloody awful sound system. The music seemed to be coming at me in waves, distorted and muted. Yet despite this the massive crowd were loving it. It appeared to me that if you wanted to get close enough to hear any of the bands properly, you had to be prepared to be crushed to death and get hit by one of the hundreds of bottles of urine that were constantly flying through the air.... lovely. Anyone who dared to venture on stage, to introduce a band, were immediately bombarded with whatever came to hand, including said bottles of pee. Brave or stupid, you decide. I settled for wandering around the stalls getting cold and miserable, ultimately making the decision to leave early and avoid the end of show chaos.

I eventually found my bike in the massive car park and headed home. I was wearing my Ashman boots under 2 pairs of jeans. My new red leather jacket, with it's heavily adorned denim waistcoat, was preparing itself to get wet as a light drizzle was starting. A blue canvas rucksack, containing something lost in memory, possibly waterproof trousers, was on my back. My bargain basement black polycarbonate helmet with it's "The Biker" magazine sticker across it's chin piece and a visor you could hardly see through was covering my non biker haircut.

It was getting dark by now but I had no idea of the time. I was fed up, cold and just wanted to get home.

After what seemed like hours on the road but clearly wasn't, the rain started to come down in torrents. I was having trouble seeing properly through the weather, and knowing that skinny Japanese tyres of that era were not exactly the most grippy of items in the wet, slowed right down to negotiate a bend in the road. The car driver behind me didn't .

I vaguely remember looking in my mirrors and seeing a Hillman Hunter behind me, getting rather too close. The next thing I knew, the bike was falling to the left.

.... now here's where physics takes over....

A motorcycle is basically a thing with two gyroscopes attached to it (wheels). Gyroscopes will naturally try and return to their original position, if forced away from it. Therefore, if left to its own devices, a motorcycle will remain upright and perfectly stable.

This is all well and good until something forces it out of that stability and it immediately tries to return to the upright position with a great deal of force, throwing off anything that is not permanently attached to it. That thing was me.

The weird thing about all of this was the feeling of total acceptance over what was about to happen. The initial rush of fear and adrenaline was replaced by a warm glow and a complete sense of weightlessness. I recall looking down on the scene below and seeing my bike resting in the gutter on it's left hand engine protection bars. I felt completely at peace until I woke up in the gutter. A lady had removed my helmet (a bit silly considering there was blood coming from under it) and had put my silk scarf under my head. "Are you alright? " she was asking.... I really didn't know.

I got scooped into an ambulance by two large chaps, with Midlands accents, and we had a nice chat on the way to hospital. I felt ok and there was no real pain but my right arm felt numb. I was almost certain it was broken.

The next thing I knew I was being undressed on a table by 3 middle aged ladies. They were very chirpy but cut off my favourite jeans with a huge pair of scissors, much to my distress.

I was examined by a doctor who started to look rather puzzled. He was asking me to move all my bits, that should move, then started to stick a pin in various parts of my right arm. He left the room, still looking puzzled and was quickly replaced by a procession of doctors with various accents, skin colour and facial expressions. The only thing they had in common, apart from the white coats and stethoscopes, was the need to stick pins in me and look as puzzled as the last one.

Eventually I was x-rayed and wheeled into a ward of groaning patients. They were nearly all attached to a multitude of traction devices and wrapped in plaster casts, some from head to toe. I got put in a bed and left overnight to worry about what the hell was going on.

My parents arrived the next morning looking more annoyed than anything. I was at the far end of the ward, so they had to walk through a scene from a bad horror movie, only to find me sat up in bed looking relatively unhurt and intact. A doctor, on his rounds, reached my bed and promptly asked who I was and what I was doing there. I told him about the accident and he asked if I could walk, I said that I thought so and got out of bed. "You can go home then." Was his final word, so I did.

My stay at the Staffordshire Royal Infirmary was one short night. Nobody seemed to know why I was there, what had happened to me or the extent of my injuries.

It transpired that I had a badly broken collarbone, my shoulder blade had been split in two, the nerves in my shoulder had been torn apart, leaving me with permanent, partial paralysis of the right arm and shoulder. My helmet had cut into my face, which needed stitches and I had a fractured spine. I still got sent home!

Apparently I had been thrown from my bike into the path of an approaching car. I hit the car, doing a fair bit of damage (according to my insurance company), bounced off the bonnet, then got run over by it.

I feel sorry for the guys in that car, merrily tootling along, only to be hit by a badly dressed, flying teenager from out of nowhere. Must have ruined their weekend.

The strangest thing about all of this is that none of it bothered me at all. There was all this drama and

mayhem going on around me and all I could think of was, *Ah well... it's happened. What now?*
No shock, no fear, no worry. The only thing that bothered me was the damage done to the front brake master cylinder on the handlebars of my bike. It ruptured during the accident, spraying brake fluid everywhere, but mostly over my, painstakingly hand painted custom, fuel tank. That did upset me a little.
My blue canvas bag had all of its buckles bent and got covered in antifreeze. I can't help but think that it took a lot of damage for me. The right shoulder of my red, Lewis Leathers jacket got ripped through two thick layers of cowhide. Undoubtedly saving my arm.

I truly believe that had I not been in the RAF when this happened and the fact that their excellent medical staff took my injuries so seriously, I would no longer have a right arm.
Ok, my shoulder doesn't work very well, if at all, and there is a loss of function in a few areas, but it's still there and most bits work fine. They sent me for all sorts of tests and even built me an arm support out of metal and leather. However, nobody actually knew how to deal with my injury.
A brachial plexus lesion is usually much more catastrophic, resulting in amputation at the

shoulder, because the arm just shrivels up and dies. I still had full use of my hand and elbow joint, albeit a little restricted. I count myself very lucky in this respect.

The RAF sent me to a joint services rehabilitation centre near London and I immediately realised just how lucky I was.

Of course my parents thought this was an end to my motorcycle stupidity.... how wrong is it possible to be ?

CHAPTER 2

'IT'S THAT ELEMENT OF SURPRISE. WHEN YOU LOSE CONTROL, YOU DISCOVER NEW THINGS.'
Daniel Lanois.

JOINT SERVICES MILITARY REHABILITATION UNIT, Somewhere near London (Secret) 1982…

It's not like I was feeling sorry for myself, not even slightly. I had to learn how to do a few things with my left arm and hand, but on the whole I was OK. Nobody was entirely sure whether I would get any use back in my shoulder but, for whatever the reason was, I wasn't that worried. The things I saw and the people I met in the rehab unit would have destroyed the most enthusiastic attempts at self pity. Some of these guys were seriously messed up.

Apart from the living consequences of various transport related mishaps and the odd freak accident, the base was populated with the results of bullets and/or shrapnel meeting human flesh and bone.

In the movies, at the time, this was usually portrayed as the victim shouting, "Ouch !" and holding the affected area whilst continuing to finish off the bad guys with a penknife. The reality is a lot more horrific, catastrophic and life changing.
This was the early 80's and the troubles in Northern Ireland were in full flow. One fellow in our barracks had been lured back to a young girl's flat, along with his buddy, only to be shot with sub machine guns, receiving 38 bullet wounds but somehow surviving. His friend was not so lucky. Officially he was dead and we were told not to tell anyone otherwise, which proved difficult because he was an arrogant, annoying little prick.

A young Military Policeman had been shot in the shin while on guard in Belfast. The shockwave from the bullet ripped out the whole of his calf muscle leaving him with just the bone to stand on. That's the thing with bullets, it's not so much the actual bullet that does any damage but the vacuum created behind it, which sucks up tissue as it travels through the body. Exit wounds are always much worse than entry wounds.
There were lots of other servicemen with various body parts missing. But these were nothing compared to the mental damage inflicted on some of these soldiers by what they had witnessed.

Despite all this, the humour, optimism and comradery throughout the place was something to behold.

I have to admit that, following my time there, I have a real problem with those disabled people who constantly whine and complain about there not being enough being done to help them or the lack of facilities, You're disabled and different, suck it up, adapt and get on with it. Accepting that there are certain things you can't do the same as everyone else is liberating.

So the World has decided you need a challenge, deal with it and make the most of what you've got. Death decided to holster his scythe and give you another chance so don't make him regret that decision.

I was put in a barrack room with a great bunch of blokes from various sections of the armed forces and in various forms of disrepair. There was even a special forces guy who was booked in as Royal Corps of Transport. He'd picked up an injury somewhere in the Middle East but it was all very 'hush hush'.

As usual, I soon made friends with the nutters in the room.

One of those nutters was known as Elvis, a name which he despised. He was my age but a throwback to the days of rockers and teddy boys. With a slicked back 'DA' hairstyle and a refusal to wear anything but black, he became my best friend on camp. He was awaiting a court martial following a fight in Berlin, which left one civilian dead and a number badly injured. He assured me that, despite what I might hear, he was very much responsible. He was there because, while on leave at his home in Lincolnshire, he was riding his old Honda CD175 motorcycle and didn't see the approaching T junction, resulting in himself and the bike jumping the bank of a drainage ditch, typical of the Lincolnshire countryside, flying across said ditch and depositing both the bike and himself on the opposite bank along with a seriously busted leg. He remained there for a total of 6 hours before he was rescued. Apparently after 2 hours, an old man walking his dog, found him and asked if he was alright. In a moment of ill advised sarcasm, Elvis replied, "Of course I'm alright mate, I do this all the time." The old man said, "Oh!.. ok then." And buggered off.

He also seemed to take great pleasure in showing me photographs of his girlfriend in studded leather bondage gear ... very odd.

When it comes to bad luck, some guys seem to have more than their fair share.

Two soldiers from the Royal Staffordshire
Regiment, both bikers, were in there together. Big
Dave and Andy.
At some point big Dave had been involved in a
minor accident while riding his Kawasaki 1300 and
ended up having a short stay in hospital. When he
was discharged, his best mate Andy went to pick
him up on his six cylinder, CBX 1000cc Honda.
On their way home, a myopic mini driver pulled
across the dual carriageway, straight in front of
them. The bike went straight through the mini,
cutting it clean in half. Needless to say they both
ended up back in hospital. The mini driver paid the
ultimate price for his carelessness and probably
didn't even know what hit him. Big Dave left most of
the flesh and muscle of his left arm on the tarmac
and suffered a head injury, which made him turn
into an uncontrollable and aggressive madman
after a couple of beers. I liked big Dave.

Perhaps the strangest case on camp was Buster.
Buster was in the Parachute Regiment and was
one of the fittest guys I've ever met. He was also
sickeningly cool.
Of mixed race, with a huge beaming smile and the
body of a Greek God, Buster could instantly charm
any girl within a 20 mile radius. This, coupled with
owning a Kawasaki Z1000 LTD custom, made him

the object of envy amongst many of the residents.
Mostly me.

'Why was he there ?' you might ask? Well,
something was seriously wrong with his
metabolism. The amount of calories Buster had to
consume was unbelievable. If he didn't, he would
simply shut down and die. His breakfast consisted
of 12 fried eggs, 6 potatoes and most of a pig. This
was just breakfast. His other meals were simply
beyond words. The most amazing part of all was
that Buster kept smiling and didn't carry a single
ounce of excess fat.

One of the few advantages of the base was that it
doubled as training centre for military chefs. The
meals were amazing and the daily menu consisted
of a choice between steak , lobster and anything
else you could imagine. The selection of deserts
could give you diabetes by just looking at them. It
was a good job that most of the day was spent in
the gym.

One day I was told to get ready for a trip to St
Thomas' hospital in London, where they could
perform some tests to find out more about the
nerve damage in my arm.

George, another biker from the Royal Tank Regiment and myself, got a chauffeur driven Ford Cortina into the city and got told to wait. We had no idea what was waiting for us. That is until I heard George screaming in pain.

When it was my turn I walked into a dark room, to find six people dressed in hospital greens. It turns out that only one would be doing the tests, the other five were there to hold me down. What followed was one of the worst experiences of my life and has left me with a great dislike of hospitals in general.

I had knitting needle size probes pushed deep into the muscles of my arm, shoulder and back to try and detect any electrical nerve impulses from my brain. It would have been better if all of my arm was dead, but it wasn't. No anaesthetic was allowed because it would have blocked the impulses. My brain has blocked and deleted a lot of memories surrounding this piece of medieval torture. All I know is that it was bloody horrible.

George's arm was found to be completely lifeless and therefore needed to be amputated. In typical army humour, all he was bothered about was that he had just spent a load of money getting his arm tattooed... what a waste.

The most important thing was that I was kept busy.

I was totally unaware that I had ADHD at the time. I don't even think such a condition existed within the medical profession's list of mental health problems. I thought it was just normal to overthink everything, lack concentration and experience everything all of the time. Ignorance is bliss, so they say.

Although this was a medical facility, it still worked like any other military establishment, with strict rules, security (perhaps more than most), inspections, etc. This regimentation and regularity suited me. It took away a lot of things that I would otherwise have to think, worry and stress about.

In the armed forces you are fed, housed, looked after medically and have no utility bills to worry about. It is no surprise to me that long serving military personnel often find it difficult to adjust to civilian life when they leave. Apart from this, it is hard to find people you can trust in 'normal' society. Having friends and colleagues that you can totally rely on, that will help and support you, no matter what, are always there in the military, but not so much on the outside. Ever wondered why so many bikers are ex forces ?

I usually spent the weekend on base, it was a lot more fun than home.

London was just a tube ride away and, on numerous visits to the capital, discovered that, despite it's huge population, people were very open and friendly. I distinctly remember buying a badge from a girl selling trinkets on the street and being amazed how talkative and chirpy she was. Maybe because she was a little strange looking, in a punk come hippy sort of way, and people seemed to avoid her, but I'm instantly drawn to that. I love the freaks, weirdos and nutcases. What is considered normal by the majority of people bores me, along with smalltalk, newspapers and the 'latest thing'. A group of us discovered a club that held a rock music event on a Thursday night, in nearby Richmond upon Thames, called The Dolphin. We'd spend the night listening to 'Juke box hero', by Foreigner, and consuming vast quantities of beer. As a result, most Friday mornings were spent hungover. Fortunately the sergeant in charge of the gym was a huge rock fan and therefore sympathetic. He also seemed to have a fondness for young men and a striking resemblance to Leslie Nielsen.

After a few long months of manipulation, correction and stretching, I was called into the camp commanding officer's office and got told that I was of no real use to the RAF with a knackered arm. It came as no surprise whatsoever. I couldn't use a rifle at the time and had a lot less mobility than I do now. He said that I could possibly stay in, but only if I became a telephonist .. Nah! Not for me thankyou. Medical discharge with exemplary, if rather short, service it was. I was sent back to RAF Cosford to be officially discharged and nearly made an officer fall off his pushbike by saluting him with my left arm. He still wasn't impressed when I explained why. Idiot.

All my personal stuff had been packed into a wooden crate and stored in a hangar.

My military life had come to an end. In some ways it came as quite a relief.

I phoned home to explain what was going on and a few days later received a letter from my father that summed him up perfectly.

Apparently I was an idiot for wanting to leave the RAF and it was all to do with 'That bunch of hippys and CND crowd'. For one, I didn't really have much of a choice, being rather badly injured and secondly, I didn't have anything to do with the CND. The man hardly ever spoke to me throughout my childhood then decides to express how he feels through a vitriolic letter. Thanks for everything Dad, great advice and support. My sincere apologies for even existing.

I think this display of fatherly love played a huge part in my getting the bike fixed as soon as possible and riding it with my arm strapped into the metal and leather brace, that the Air Force medical boffins created for me. Perhaps not really advisable but anything that got me out of that house was worth it.

All I needed was a new job, some new friends, and a few cans of spray paint.

I had nothing to do at home, which is a recipe for chaos in my head.

I started fiddling around with the bike, replacing the scratched silencers with offensively loud, 70's style trumpet items and tried numerous handlebar options, from high and wide to low and narrow race style. The latter resulting in the throttle sticking open due to poor cable routing, rapid twitching of the sphincter and thankfulness for the kill switch. Handlebars have been a constant problem since damaging my shoulder and finding exactly the right riding position has been both a challenge and an excuse for changing my motorcycle so many times. The real reason is that I was constantly searching for something new, something different and something faster.

Whenever I found another bike, it was only a matter of time before things started getting messed about with, painted or changed. I believe I must have

been the first biker in the UK to have luminous pink
wheels. Not sure if I'm proud of that or not ?
I started to paint the petrol tank on the 250, using
spray cans to create a mural of the Pied Piper. I got
the idea from a Jethro Tull song of the same name,
but It looked bloody awful and never got finished.
The poor bike started to look a mess.
Time was running out for me being able to ride the
Suzuki on 'L' plates. The new learner laws were
drawing closer and, if I didn't pass my bike test
soon, I would be forced to ride a 125cc machine. I
really didn't fancy that.
I attended a motorcycle training course, just to
make sure I didn't make any stupid mistakes on my
test. It paid off. I passed my test, despite my brake
light sticking on, with just a few weeks to go before
the law changed.

I was out of work so made my way to the Job
Centre in Chester. They immediately decided that I
was disabled, issued me with a green card to prove
it and sent me to see the relevant advisor. They
were most helpful to be fair and suggested that I
might like to go to Preston, to a specialised centre
that would assess my ability to work and find out
what I could or couldn't do. It turns out there was
nothing I couldn't do and that I was pretty damn
good at most things I could.

Apart from working on things that need both arms raised above my head, anything was possible. I discovered that I could take a car engine apart and rebuild it, I wasn't bad at welding and I could make an electric doorbell from a circuit diagram. The best thing about the centre was that it was full of crazy people. I felt very much at home.

Preston has to be one of the friendliest towns I have ever spent time in. The people there were great and naturally friendly, especially the biker community who congregated at the Dog and Partridge pub in the town centre.

The establishment was run by a gay, ex police officer who, unlike many landlords of that era, welcomed us scruffy bunch of hooligans with open arms. The pub was divided into 2 similar but distinctly separate areas. The back of the pub was what I referred to as the hard-core section. I was a rather skinny 20 year old at the time and the guys in this section were somewhat intimidating, but nonetheless fascinating. Anyone who inadvertently wandered into that area usually found themselves outside in the back yard, on their arses, with not much idea of how they got there and with some part of their anatomy smarting a little. Yet, if you showed these guys a bit of respect, they would help you out with anything.

It was here that I was introduced to the world of motorcycle clubs and was soon a member of the, creatively named, Dog and Partridge MCC (MotorCycle Club).

To be quite honest, we didn't do much… apart from drink a lot.

Back at the centre I had become friends with Ted, he was around my age but looked more like an 80 year old. He hailed from deepest, darkest, rural Shropshire, near Lydbury North (sound familiar?). Due to badly mangling his leg in a bike accident, he rode around on a Honda 400 four with a small white sidecar attached. I spent many an enjoyable evening cruising around Preston in that sidecar, wearing a peaked woolen beanie hat and aviator goggles. I have to admit spending a small percentage of that time with my eyes shut and silently praying to any gods that might be listening, but it was great fun all the same.

I was still not confident, or fit enough to ride my Suzuki 250 up to Preston. There was a guy by the name of Gordon (yes, he was a bit of a moron) who lived in Chester and claimed to have ridden every bike in existence. In hindsight I rather foolishly agreed to let him ride my bike up to Preston with myself riding pillion. Bad mistake.

It was a pleasant Sunday afternoon, on the Northbound M6 motorway, and we were happily buzzing along in the outside lane, overtaking slower moving traffic. When suddenly the outside lane slowed almost to a standstill. We didn't!

Gordon the moron didn't stop quickly enough and we ended up hitting the bumper of the car in front. Not so hard that any real damage was done to either vehicle but the laws of gravity dictated that we fell off. Unfortunately the impact, although minimal, had caused the drive chain to come of it's sprockets, hit the clutch pushrod and break the oil seal. This meant that when the bike was restarted, the resultant oil pressure spewed a jet of engine oil onto the motorway tarmac.

We pushed the bike onto the hard shoulder and could soon hear the approaching sound of a police vehicle. I expected the worst but it turned out that the copper could not have been more helpful. He didn't even ask any questions or want to see any documents. He just escorted myself and a dribbling Suzuki 250 off the motorway, with my hand hovering over the clutch in case the engine seized. I limped into the garage of the rehab centre and began my, self taught, crash course in motorcycle mechanics and how to swear a lot.

On reflection I think it's fair to say that I didn't have a clue what I was doing. Not just mechanically but with my life in general. I had no idea that my brain was wired differently than most people. I had no thoughts about the future and was just living day to day. Once again I was housed, fed and watered, with not a care in the World.

I fixed the bike by myself and, despite my injury, realised that with a little planning and adaptation, there wasn't much that I couldn't achieve. Including taking an engine out of a motorcycle and putting it back in when it was fixed.

There is always a way around things, perhaps in a slightly unorthodox manner with a slight hint of ridiculousness, but always a way. It's also very rewarding, especially if somebody suggests that I can't do it on my own.

The clientele of the establishment for the broken and bewildered varied a great deal. Some were there due to injury, some through illness and others through self inflicted bodily abuse.

One such fellow, whose name escapes me, occupied a 6 man room by himself. There was a bed for him and the rest of the space was taken up by huge boxes of fluid. I'm not really sure what the fluid was but he had to attach said boxes to a tap in his abdomen and sit still for hours. He'd managed to severely mess up his body with a huge variety of mind altering chemicals and those boxes were the only thing keeping him alive.

He asked a few of us to call by his room one night and, on opening his door, were greeted by a thick green haze of cannabis smoke.

I've never really bothered much with cannabis, mainly because I don't like smoking, but after a few minutes in that room, I was not feeling fully in touch with terra firma and started grinning for no apparent reason.

Despite what had happened to this guy, he showed no signs of wanting to change his ways. His life, his choice.

My ever searching and wandering mind often made me think about drugs and what they did, but to be quite honest, I have rarely felt the need. My brain is more than capable of creating it's own fantasies, parallel universes and hallucinations on it's own. Synapses are in overdrive for most of my day and I'm an expert in amusing myself, if nobody else. However I was a little curious and one Friday evening a bag full of dried magic mushrooms appeared. They were pretty disgusting to eat, a bit like eating dry grass, but after my stomach had made sense of them and broken them down into something digestible, the psilocybin made it's way to my grey matter. The most noticeable effect was that my brain went strangely quiet. This is possibly what most people's brains feel like but not mine. It may well have been this silence that brought about the feeling of euphoria, I couldn't really say. It felt good.

I hadn't eaten a huge amount so the effects were not too dramatic. I do recall sitting there watching TV with four of my friends and nearly wetting ourselves laughing at what we saw. Not unusual apart from the fact that it was a chat show about politics, but the boring faces of each politician, who were being very serious indeed, were absolutely hilarious. Then we made the mistake of looking at each other… we were even funnier.

I finally decided to retire to my room, but discovered that my feet would not make contact with the floor. It felt like I was walking six inches above the ground. How I found the right door must have been sheer luck. I finally made it to my bed and lay there contemplating why the walls were made of chocolate and where I could find some more mushrooms.

I was spending a lot more of my spare time at the Dog and Partridge. I felt comfortable there, amongst like minded folk, cheap beer, and an excellent juke box.

Being rather shy and lacking self confidence meant that my experiences with regard to the fairer sex were limited to being forced to sit next to Cheryl Baker at school, as a punishment for talking, and finding out she was actually pretty cool. The rest was down to a lot of imagination and the magazines I found in my father's bedside cupboard. What I had definitely never experienced was a girl approaching me and striking up a conversation, it simply didn't happen to me. This seemed quite the norm in Preston however and usually left me with general paralysis, my ability to speak deserting me and bursting into a cold sweat.

On one occasion I was accosted by a truly beautiful young girl outside the pub. Her mate had been hanging around Gordon the moron for a while and she had taken a shine to me. At the time she epitomized all that I could have ever dreamt of in a girl. Long blond hair that reached right down to her hips, legs poured into tight blue jeans and huge pale blue eyes. I managed to talk to her without making a complete idiot out of myself and went into the pub to buy us both a drink. I ordered two pints and was asked by the barman who the other drink was for. When I explained who it was, he refused to serve me due to the fact that the blonde goddess sitting outside was only 15 years old. Just my luck.

I had developed a taste for Stones bitter by now and if I wasn't riding, would manage about 4 pints and just the one if I was. One evening I must have been enjoying myself more than usual and got through a whole lot more. I had arrived on the bike but thought that I would push it into the backyard of the pub where it would be safe (common practice for this fine establishment.), but as I got steadily more inebriated, decided that I'd be fine to ride it home and proceeded to do so in the pouring rain. To this day I have no idea how I managed to ride the bike or navigate the 4 miles back to the garage, but I did. I had drank around 12 pints and swore to myself that I would never drink and ride again. Stupid, stupid, stupid.
On a side note; I have kept this promise.

With the bike fully functional, a new found knowledge of how it worked and still no idea what I would do next, the time came for me to go home to Chester. I was not looking forward to it at all. Over the past 3 years I had learnt a lot about life, people, and that there was a lot more to life than what living with my parents had to offer.

Home life was like being in a prison where nobody talked to me and it felt like I was just in the way. I wanted to do everything all at once but I was going to get very bored again, and that's never a good thing.

I didn't know what I was going to do with myself. I just knew that I had to leave home as soon as I could.

CHAPTER 3

'You start the game with a full pot o' luck and an empty pot o' experience. The object is to fill the pot of experience before you empty the pot of luck.'
Unknown.

Vicars Cross, Chester, 1970 something…
'Must try harder', 'Has a tendency to daydream', 'A polite and pleasant student but can do better', etc, etc.
Every school year my report was put in an envelope for me to gingerly pass to my parents. On the plus side they actually took notice of their pale, quiet offspring.
The report could have said anything as far as I was concerned. I had other things on my mind, a million other things, and that was the problem.

I always had another million things to do, usually while I was trying to finish something else (this still happens a lot).
With this constant need to be busy came an even bigger need to receive some sort of affirmation that what I was doing was right, or simply that I had done it well.

I think, partly due to the complete lack of understanding or any sort of encouragement and support from my, somewhat distant, parents, I would often find myself up to mischief with varying degrees of danger.

With the gift of hindsight, I suppose I would often hope to get caught, just so that it would elicit some sort of attention. Alas this was rarely the case and it just spurred me into further acts of stupidity and danger.

My swirling mind took on the form of an imaginary friend and partner in mischief, Johnny. Although not real, it must be said that he had some brilliant ideas.

Perhaps the best being 6 feet long garden cane, tomato launchers that would launch tomatoes high into the air and plummet down to earth somewhere out of sight, splattering onto a, thoroughly confused, local resident's patio or greenhouse. Probably no more confused than a mother wondering who was eating so many tomatoes.

However not all of Johnny's ideas were so clever, especially the ones involving a box of matches and wax floor polish, or those involving local building sites.

The latter were the most fun, especially after the discovery that if you stuck the end of a small piece of copper pipe into a bag of cement and flicked it towards your chosen target, it would send a pellet of concrete powder out of the end like a bullet. Returning home covered head to toe in grey dust, trying to deny that I had been anywhere near the building site, was never going to end well. Apart from that, my mother worked behind the counter of our local Post Office, so she had spies everywhere.

Looking back, I often wonder how I managed to stay out of hospital or do some permanent damage to myself. I waited until I was 19 years old to do that.

My brain chatter never stops except for a few, rare exceptions. Once was when I tried an ecstasy tablet in the early 90's. This was the first time that I had ever experienced total, mental peace. It was like a cold wave rushed through my brain and switched off everything apart from what I wanted to hear. I felt like I was wrapped in a cocoon of warm sunshine and everything was good with the World. Music took on a whole new meaning and I felt thoroughly content.
It was this event that confirmed to my psychiatrist that I had been living with ADHD throughout my life. The second time was when I had an out of body

experience, following my motorcycle accident in 1981 (aged 19). I felt myself flying weightlessly through the darkness, completely devoid of brain chatter, worries or fear and looking down at my crashed bike, lying on it's side in the gutter. When I had my bike returned to me I knew exactly how and where it had been damaged. I believe it must have been a near death experience.

The closest I came to finding peace, prior to these events, was when I took up fishing as a child. Sitting in the countryside, by a pond, in the summertime, may seem like the perfect place for an overactive brain to go wild. However, concentrating on that tiny float, looking for bites, focused the mind perfectly. Problems occurred after an hour or so if nothing happened and I resorted to climbing the nearest tree, skimming stones or running around the field naked.
If I went fishing with friends, we'd end up having cow shit fights if nobody was catching anything. That took some explaining to my mother also.

Without a doubt the best therapy for anyone living with ADHD is music. Everyone has their own particular taste in music but for me it was mostly rock.

With the help of my local library, where I could borrow the latest vinyl LPs, I discovered bands like Pink Floyd, Led Zeppelin, Hawkwind and Deep Purple. The intensity, passion and song content immediately appealed to me and I was hooked. People find it difficult to understand how listening to Lamb of God, a very intense thrash metal band, can help me drift off to sleep, but there is so much going on within the music that it leaves no room for anything else to creep into my mind and it deeply relaxes me.

I am never without music, there is a backing track to everything I do, from the second I wake up until I go to sleep. I always wake up with a random song in my head, even ones I don't like very much.

I can mentally playback songs I know, note for note and compose new tunes in my head.

You would think that I would be an accomplished musician by now but I quickly got bored whenever I tried to learn how to play an instrument. If it didn't make a tune immediately, I gave up. So nowadays I sing, it's not like I can put my voice away to gather dust in the attic.

I was stuck at home again with a father that seemed to be in a state of permanent, simmering angst and a mother that seemed perfectly happy about it.

As for myself, there was an overwhelming need for a bigger, faster motorcycle to provide more adrenaline buzz or street cred, imagined or otherwise. Most of all I needed some sort of mental stimulus. It was time to look for another machine. Alas, I was somewhat financially embarrassed and, due to the new laws, which meant learner riders were only able to ride a 125cc machine, I was left with a bike nobody wanted to buy. Needless to say, as I'm certain happened with a number of 250cc motorcycles of the early 1980's, it suddenly went missing. Perhaps it was abducted by extraterrestrials for experimentation and anal probing, then dropped back to Earth, which provided an excellent explanation as to why it was found semi-submerged in a pond about 10 miles from my house.

Of course I have no idea how this happened, but I ended up with a rather pitiful payout from my insurance company, which barely paid off the remaining finance, and went in search of some new wheels, in my hyperactive, impetuous and impatient manner.

Back then there wasn't a great deal to choose from, if you were lacking in funds, out of work and couldn't get a loan.

Old British bikes needed a fully equipped workshop, just to keep them running and an endless supply of oil. It was also quite obvious that there was no way I was ever going to be able to afford a brand new Japanese model or even a decent second hand one from a dealership.

Seeing as this was to be my only form of transport, I needed something solid and reliable. It also had to look the part, obviously.

During the first part of the 1980s it was a lot simpler to shop for a motorcycle because there wasn't such a huge selection to choose from. I didn't want anything too big and powerful because I wasn't sure whether I could handle a larger capacity machine, let alone afford to buy or insure one. I was left travelling in circles around the local dealers in a fruitless search for a piece of mechanical mediocrity which would satisfy my longings and display a price tag that didn't make me sigh in despair.

It was around this time that I began to realise that being without a motorcycle felt like losing a limb. I found it really difficult to get along without one.

They had become part of my existence, personality and very soul.

I had recently become part of a local motorcycle club called the Evicted MCC. Their name deriving from being kicked out of the Boathouse pub, on the banks of the river in Chester, when the owners decided that bikers were non-desirables and did not fit in with their image of a trendy riverside establishment.

Their new home was in a particularly untrendy but very welcoming, hostelry on the outskirts of Chester, known as the Lock Vaults, which was, unsurprisingly, next to a canal. A pint of mild ale was 50 pence, it had a decent jukebox, a space invaders machine and most importantly it put up with us lot. It was also within walking or wobbling distance of home.

I would struggle along to rallys and events on my little 250 and it never let me down, even carrying a passenger, military tent (which weighed more than the passenger) and luggage, up the motorway in freezing conditions to a pub near Bolton (I think). We set up camp on the frost covered bowling green then proceeded to blank out the cold with the aid of alcohol... as per normal.

My fondest memory of this particular rally was Chris. I have yet to see anyone shit, puke and pee all at the same time since this incredible achievement. The stuff of legends.

Our tent developed a frozen river through the middle of it and everywhere had a thick, white blanket of frost clinging to it, but we cared not. We were hard-core... or just plain nuts. Probably the latter. I had my first ever experience of a vindaloo curry, bought from a nearby take away. It had the texture of wet sand, but is was very hot and probably stopped me becoming hypothermic. Winter rallies were commonplace back then and were great because all the idiots stayed at home (apart from us of course). It was where you could meet up with all the other rally nutters. You'd see the same old faces on filthy bikes, because they were too busy being ridden to get washed. There were no bands playing, unless it was a local folk band, there was just a field, beer and some drunken singing. Oh !... There were silly games too.

I have nearly died twice. Once when I was knocked of my bike and the second time was during one of those silly games.

Most of these games involved eating, drinking, tug of war or throwing something. On this particular occasion the item being thrown was a ship's piston, with conrod attached. A huge thing that was hard enough to lift, let alone throw. The preferred technique appeared to be rotating like a hammer thrower then releasing It at just the right moment, sending it gracefully down the field. That is unless your name is Matty.

His rotations started well and things were looking good for an Evicted victory, until a slight backwards stumble, from our resident strongman, caused a premature release of this rusty lump of maritime mechanics into orbit. On seeing this, the crowd scattered. I ran with the others, wondering when and where the space bound projectile would re-enter the atmosphere and crash to Earth. I soon found out. It was via my, already damaged right shoulder, only fractionally missing my head and certain, but probably quite painless, death. Never mind eh? I was so cold that I barely felt a thing and carried on drinking.

When I think back to those days, one character from the Evicted crowd stands out in my memory. George.
If I thought my mind was a little hyperactive, George's was in a league of its own. This guy slept with his eyes open. Literally. Quite disturbing when you've been talking to him for the last quarter of an hour.
He owned a bright red Norton Commando 750 that only had a front brake. It actually did have a back brake aswell, but it was so covered in oil from leaks in the engine, as to render it useless.

Our Saturday night pub crawls would always end up at George's house. As soon as we arrived, he'd put on old Rolling Stones record on the player and leave it on repeat. He bore in uncanny resemblance to a young Mick Jagger. So much so that it lead to many of us questioning whether or not he could have been an illegitimate son of the randy rock star. My usual trick on such nights, was to start feeling a bit wobbly, sneak out of the door and wobble the 3 miles home.

I was gradually becoming aware that alcohol could bring a certain degree of calm to my racing mind. Unfortunately I often got to a point where I would lose sight of the stop sign and end up depositing whatever I had consumed and imbibed down the toilet or in the corner of a field (the first time consisting of many pints of bitter mixed with 3 plates of hot pot at the 'Boots and Saddles' rally, somewhere near Chorley in Lancashire).

I think that many of us who suffer from ADD/ADHD find comfort in mind altering substances. It is a dangerous route to follow and can easily lead to addiction or dependence. Thankfully I have managed to avoid this road, so there must be something in there that knows when to stop, or an overworked guardian angel watching over me.

Perhaps too many post rally, hungover, Sunday wobbles home with a thumping headache and a mouth like the bottom of a poorly hamster's cage have taught me that lesson.

What I like most about biker events is that pretty much everyone there respects each other. Yes, there are occasions when things get out of hand, but they are self policing by their very nature.
In 1986 I was one of 26,000 bikers attending a well known event in the South East of England. The police presence consisted of two constables, one male the other female, who were just wandering around enjoying a bit of easy overtime. They were simply not required and there was little or no trouble. If there was, it was dealt with most effectively by the event organisers.
I must add here that anyone who doesn't believe in the devil, has never been to a large biker event or festival. Those little blue rows of temporary toilets, especially on a Saturday or Sunday morning, are portals to Hell itself. It becomes a case of picking the one least likely to leave you with dysentary or cholera. If there's a queue, then it becomes a horrific lottery.
I've no idea what happens in there at times. It's as if a grizzly bear has been out drinking Guinness all night, had 5 Indian takeaways and downed a

catering tin of prunes for desert. Even then it must
have performed some kind of break dance routine
whilst emptying it's bowels.
If at all possible they are best being avoided, unless
you're lucky enough to get there just after they've
been emptied and cleaned. During particularly hot
spells they become like mini ovens, cooking and
fermenting whatever has been deposited inside.
They truly are little blue capsules of delight.

I cannot emphasise enough how important that
word 'Respect' is to the biker community. It binds
us together and sets us apart from the rest of
society.
We help and support each other. We consider the
feelings and needs of our brothers and sisters. We
never judge or look down upon others and,
regardless of anything, treat each other as equals.
Amongst fellow bikers is one of the few places
where I can fully relax. I find it difficult to feel fully at
ease in any other public place. I know that there are
a lot of good people out there, who are not part of
my World, but I err on the side of caution. So if I
count you as a friend, you must be rather special
and mean a great deal to me.
I don't regard myself as something special, above
you, or your better... quite the opposite in fact.
I spend every waking hour questioning myself and

never feel that I am being or doing enough. It is almost impossible to totally relax with a mind that runs without a buffer. It's like living in an airport departure lounge on a bank holiday weekend but 24/7, with 10 backing tracks and 20 video screens playing random tracks and images at full volume. When I ride my motorcycle I have to focus or I will be in trouble. This focus brings me mental peace.

Anyway… I was still bikeless and feeling crap because of it.
On perusal of the local newspaper's for sale section, it jumped out at me (mostly because it didn't cost much). Just a few miles away was a 1976 model Suzuki GT 380.
In the 1970's, Suzuki decided it would be a great idea to produce a range of 2 stroke, 3 cylinder tourers... a bit of a contradiction in itself but they were actually rather nice machines. There was a choice of 3 models at the time.
A totally insane GT 750 triple with ridiculous power, chassis and brakes that were next to useless, when coupled with this screaming banshee of an engine and the nickname 'kettle', due to it being water cooled.
It's little brother was an air cooled 550cc triple, and then there was the runt of the litter, the GT 380.

With three cylinders, amazing build quality, a very comfy seat and it's own pale blue smoke screen. It ticked all the boxes for me, so I phoned the guy and was at his house within 20 minutes.

Apart from the fact that one of the bike's ignition coils had been replaced by one off an Austin Mini and clamped to the frame didn't bother me at all. I was overwhelmed by my need to be on two wheels again and had already decided to buy it regardless. It was a decent looking machine overall. I replaced the coils with a set from a breakers yard and fitted some S&B air filters, that created a very pleasing, hollow, throaty roar as air was being sucked into the 3 carburettors. Considering it was only 380cc, it was pretty nippy, even with a passenger. So much so, that at the junction of George Street and Northgate Street in Chester, it was not unusual for me to get airborne, depending on whether the traffic lights were in my favour.

If I could ever get back any of the multitude of motorcycles from my youth, this would be it. I named her Doris and loved her to bits. But as per normal, I still wanted more. Ho hum ....

I had drifted away from my parents completely, they didn't feel like family at all, more like strangers that tolerated somebody else living in their home.

My siblings had all flown the nest as soon as they could.

My eldest brother had joined the merchant navy and was travelling the globe, my sister had got married and moved in with her husband and my other brother had joined the army at 15 to escape the tension of our strange household. It was only much later in my life that I found out why and it wasn't very nice.

Between my closest sibling and myself, there is an 11 year gap, which has always left me thinking that I might have been a mistake, or maybe just something to keep my mother busy. One thing I have yet to figure out is that when I was only a year old, my mother took me on a flight across the Atlantic (a huge undertaking in 1963) to visit the mother of an American soldier that she had been seeing during the war. She had kept in touch with her, in her remote little house, located rural in West Virginia, since her son , called DUANE (the name that she chose for me), was sent back to the USA after the second world war.

Why on earth would you go through a trip like that, with a very small child, on your own, to see the mother of an ex boyfriend, while your husband stays at home? Perhaps it's just me that finds the whole thing rather peculiar, but let's be honest, it's weird.

Our family home in Vicars Cross, on the outskirts of Chester, held many strange and unexplainable memories for me.

There was one particular room in which I spent most of my time. I would draw pictures of mythical creatures, build Airfix models and listen to music on a huge 'stereogram'. This was known as the dining room and boasted a large black marble fireplace, which always seemed a little out of place.

I had been left home alone, at age 15, while the folks went away on holiday, abroad somewhere. I was just on my way to bed and, for some reason, decided to check my favourite room, just in case I had left anything electrical switched on. As I pushed the door, it opened about 10 inches then violently slammed shut as if pushed from inside. I was alone, it was dark and I very nearly pooped myself. I ran upstairs and hid under my blankets, too scared to move.

Another time was when I decided to lie down on my bed for a quick nap. It was one of those not quite asleep but not quite awake, fuzzy headed sort of naps, and just as I was coming out of that semi conscious state, felt the whole, feet end, of the bed crash back down to the floor after it had risen off the ground by about 6 inches.

There was also a ghostly cat, who would often jump

onto my bed. You couldn't see it, but felt it walking across your legs and pawing the bedclothes. Quite soothing in a strange sort of way.

It doesn't end with the house. I don't know if it's due to my permanently switched on brain, but I feel energy very strongly.

I noticed this at quite an early age when I was always drawn to Chester Cathedral. A beautiful building with an amazing history dating back to the 9th century.... and I certainly felt it !!! Whenever I walked through the doors my whole body would be filled with, what I can only describe as, static electricity. I would be literally buzzing inside. This has never left me and I don't want it to. I can pick up on energy anywhere that has any, but take me to a known haunted location and I may as well be plugged into the mains. The big difference on such occasions is that I see things that others simply cannot. That's when it gets really interesting.

I see figures traced out by tiny electrical discharges like tiny lightning bolts. It's just a case of allowing the mind to accept such things as a reality and there you go. I have witnessed such figures in many places and I have often found myself going for the brakes when a figure crosses the road in front of me, only for them to disappear into the ether. This happens regularly and I'm getting used to it.

I recall riding along a quiet road one night and noticing a fellow riders headlamp appear in my mirrors, just a few feet behind me. It's always good to ride with a fellow soul, so I thought nothing of it. That is until the light just vanished. There were no junctions or properties along that stretch of road where they could have gone and I turned around to check if anything had happened, but no. Poof!
 Gone.
But I digress.... as is so often the case.

The thing about bikes for me *is* their energy. Everything has it but most can't feel it. If you embrace and connect with that energy it pays you back in kind. I don't get on a motorcycle and ride it, I become part of it. It becomes an extension of myself and every little movement, sound and feeling flows through me.
I consider myself to be a follower of Buddhist ways. Not by wearing orange robes and chanting, but the whole attitude. Buddhists believe that everything has a 'soul' and has a purpose. Because of this, anything that is created for a purpose already knows what it is supposed to do. Therefore you have to just let it do it's thing. Attempting to force it to do otherwise will just end badly. A bit like telling someone to be happy, *or else.*
A motorcycle is no different. If you were not meant

to be together, or you treat it disrespectfully, it won't be long before it lets you know. It happened when I sold one of my bikes to someone in a future chapter.

Everything in your life has a voice, it's just that people choose not to listen anymore.
Yeah OK.. I'm a weirdo but it works for me.

CHAPTER 4

*'Every person with ADHD already knows that
destination addiction is part of their disorder.
However, if it doesn't have a positive outlet, it can
destroy your life. It is not another person that will
make your life better; it is the qualities in them that
you admire. Incorporate those attributes into your
own life and you won't miss a thing.'*
— **Shannon L. Alder**

A transparent plastic box in the shape of the
number 3, filled with dead leaves.
An orang utan.
Some Mr Kiplings fondant fancies.
A porcelain clown.
'Monkey Man' by Toots and the Maytals.
Why did John Lennon marry Yoko Ono ?
Snails....

Confused? Don't worry, they're in my head not
yours. Along with a million other images, ideas,
thoughts and scenarios with their own soundtrack.
All day, every day.
It's happening when I'm watching TV, reading a
book, attempting to sleep, and when you're talking
to me.

Since I can remember, this has been the case and
until last year, at the age of 54, I thought it was the
same for everyone. It would appear not.
The man sitting opposite me, with fingers
interlocked in front of him and a clipboard on his
lap, tells me I've been living with my close and

enthusiastic friend, ADHD, since birth.

It isn't all bad though. When you are completely unaware that something is wrong, it becomes normality. Growing up in the 1960's and 70's meant that nobody else was aware of the condition anyway, so I was just left to cope inside my own little bubble of daydreams and imagination. To be quite honest, I had a great time.

School only became a problem for me when we were wrenched from the hands of dinner ladies and taken away from sandpits and finger paints, with the intention that we should start learning something.
If a subject was of no interest to me or didn't thoroughly engage me, it just became part of the ever present background noise, until I was snapped out my dream state by a ruler being slammed on my desk or the chalk dust clouded, sharp pain as a blackboard eraser ricocheted off my head.
Yet an over busy brain is a naturally creative brain and I excelled at art, even though some teachers didn't quite understand some of my creations.
Never needing anything to copy from, I had enough ideas to keep the biggest gallery supplied for an eternity. It was a pity that other subjects got in the way.
Towards the end of junior school, it finally dawned upon my parents that I might be struggling a little, or perhaps just stupid.
Our teacher was a hippy who didn't teach us much at all, not that it would have made much difference to me. We used to spend lesson times pretending to be the band 'The Sweet' and perform 'Ballroom

Blitz' on a regular basis. I was the singer, Brian Connolly.

I really wasn't lacking intelligence, just the ability to concentrate. It only really became an issue when a new, psychopathic, teacher took over our class. Mr Owen would be locked away in a padded cell nowadays. This bespectacled, tight collared, red faced lunatic thought nothing of hitting 10 year old kids and punched me in the chest when I had the audacity to glance out of the window. My father and this raving nutcase seemed to hit it off right away and the next thing I knew I was sat down in front of the entrance exam for the King's School. A posh private school on the outskirts of Chester for particularly brainy kids. I had a better chance of going 10 rounds against Muhammed Ali and winning on points than passing the exam. I don't think I could answer a single question.

The next attempt to save me from unsuccessfulness, was to try and get me into Chester Cathedral Choir School.... *what the hell*?

I had to sing a song, that I had never heard before, in front of an odd looking old bloke at a piano. I had never sang in front of anyone, ever. Fortunately I was nowhere near good enough. It actually scares me to think about what that would have done to me. Years of bible classes and inappropriate behaviour from my smock wearing tutors I imagine. Scary.

I understand that he, possibly, had my (or more likely his) best interests in mind, but all this achieved was to further convince both him and myself that I was bloody useless and a complete failure.

I ended up, with everyone else that didn't pass the 11 plus exam and make it to grammar school, with the rest of the local 'not quite brainy enoughs' at our local secondary school.

Perhaps due to father's masonic connections, I was put into the top class. I was the youngest in the class (my birthday was just as we broke up for summer holidays). I was seriously lacking in academic ability and surrounded by a collection of highly intelligent, conscientious and confident aliens. I started drowning immediately.

Blessed with ears that stuck out like jug handles, no interest in anything that anyone else seemed to be 'into' and a complete lack of social skills, I began 5 years of hell.

I had my hair set on fire on the school bus, regular public humiliations by various teachers and got told to 'run it off' and made to throw a discus after I broke my wrist during sports class.

I remember being called into the headmasters office. This had only happened once before, when myself and Andrew Green had been reported for throwing empty drink cans onto the road, to watch them get squashed by cars, which resulted in getting caned across the fingers. I imagine it had something to do with father's masonic connections, once again, that Mr George (known as Judder to us schoolkids) suggested that I might like to become a jeweller's assistant. I mean, where did this shit come from?

I sometimes think I must have slipped into another dimension, either that, or the most likely reason, that I had parents who didn't have the tiniest idea or interest in what their youngest son was doing or wanted to do. They never even asked. Just presumed.

I wasn't stupid or disruptive at school, in truth I was a total nerd with sticky out ears, poor dress sense (it was the 70's after all) and got picked on all the time because I was a bit of a wimp. I used to spend most break times in the library or doing project work, just to avoid the bullying, imagined or otherwise. If I witness bullying nowadays, the red mist descends, but looking back I feel sorry for those lads that used to pick on me. Most of them were from homes where domestic violence was the norm. It was their way of fighting back and letting off steam.

The whole experience was pretty much summed up when Mr Armitage brought the school goat into class and it emptied it's bladder onto my canvas school bag.

I hated every second I had to spend in that school. I had much more interesting things to be doing.

None of them educationally based activities.

For some reason, probably a random idea, I decided to join the Air Cadets. This was undoubtedly the best thing I had ever done.

In that mini air force, I found some great friends and something to occupy my thoughts.

There were a couple of officers looking after the rabble. One was the Commanding Officer of the squadron, a really pleasant, elderly gentleman, with nothing but the welfare of us all in mind. Then there was the Flying Officer.

We nicknamed him 'Peachy', I can't remember why but he was a bit of a dick. I don't know why he was even there. He did nothing but ridicule and torment us all while strutting around, wearing aviator shades or driving his Triumph TR7. On the plus side, he taught me how to ski by dragging me up to the top of a mountain in Italy and telling me there was only one way down. It worked.

All of us used to be struck dumb by his wife. She was absolutely gorgeous, in a 70's kind of way. She single handedly fuelled our adolescent fantasies and kept Kleenex in business for a number of years.

The strangest fellow was the Squadron Warrant Officer. He spoke in a very high pitched voice and couldn't be taken seriously when giving orders or squeaking drill commands.

He used to be part of the hospital radio staff at, what is now known as, The Countess of Chester Hospital. On various evenings during the week he would invite a select few of the cadets to join him and help out. I didn't bother because of what the other lads were telling me about it. It was eventually discovered that there were some very odd things going on there of a sexual nature and there was a reason why he liked being involved with young boys. Dirty old git. I believe he eventually got prosecuted for his perverted behaviour.

The best thing about the Space Cadets (as I chose to call them) was getting scared shitless on a Sunday morning, flying around in gliders at RAF Sealand. This involved getting airborne by the use of a high speed winch, which resulted in a more or less vertical ascent. Floating above the steelworks in an open cockpit. Then having just one chance to make it back to Earth in the right place and in one piece. It was a massive adrenaline rush.

It was being an air cadet that made me decide to join the Royal Air Force and it helped a great deal when it came to basic training. I already knew how to look after my uniform, what to do on the drill square, how to handle a rifle and, most of all, how to get along in a squad of nutcases and reprobates whilst being shouted at. It was a breeze.

Back in the early 1980's I was blissfully unaware that my brain was wired differently. Nobody even knew that ADD/ADHD was even a thing. Things only come into existence if they get named or labelled, which is not always a good thing.
I was living day to day with no plans, no worries and no idea what was going on. I had moved out of the parental home because, after spending so much time away in the Royal Air Force, I just couldn't face the deafening silence and tension that was constantly simmering away in that emotionless house.
I was living near Chester city centre, just down the road from the Renegades MC clubhouse, a 1% motorcycle club (Google it), as well as a smattering of bikers along the street, which seemed to be made up of bedsits and student accommodation.
I had moved in with my girlfriend at the time and her family, far from ideal but it was away from what never really felt like home.
Having absolutely nothing but silence, interrupted by a lot of 'tutting', to base a relationship upon, I had no idea what was the right thing to do or how to act.
If my parents ever showed each other the tiniest piece of love or affection they kept it very well hidden. They mostly just sat in silence, sipping cups of tea.
As a child I used to look on in wonder at other families and how they got along. It was like they were from a completely different universe to mine. Apart from anything else, they actually spoke to

each other and had fun. Did things together and enjoyed each other's company.

I used to wonder how other guys managed to find a girlfriend. They seemed to have no problem talking to a girl and, more often than not, end up going home with them.
Myself, in the meantime, would just sit there scared to even smile at a member of the opposite sex. My mind would create so many negative scenarios that I had already accepted a total rejection before the girl was aware that I even existed.
To say that I was awkward would be a huge understatement. As far as I was concerned there was a huge neon sign above my head that read 'Hopeless Wanker'. The sad thing is that, by all accounts, quite a few girls actually really fancied me, but I never dared imagine that this was the case. If they smiled at me I thought they were laughing and if they ever spoke to me I wouldn't know what to say. I would blush redder than the setting sun and break into a cold sweat. It wasn't like I was ugly either. I had hair half way down my back, blue eyes, a slim physique and generally looked ok, but my confidence and self esteem were lower than a daschund's bollocks in deep snow.
I recall an occasion when a gorgeous looking girl, wearing a very tight, black mini dress, started dancing, in a very sexy and provocative manner, right in front of me. My mate was nudging me and it was obvious what was on offer. I just sat there dumbstruck, afraid to even look her in the eye.
Some 35 years later, apart from the hair, nothing much has changed.
Despite my debilitating awkwardness, I had somehow managed to get myself a girlfriend.

Can't really remember exactly how it happened.
She must have been desperate.

The disability advisor guy at the Job Centre
decided that I should put in for a job working as a
data input clerk for our local electricity supplier. It
turned out to be my idea of hell on Earth.
It was based in a huge multi storied edifice that
looked like a three legged starfish from above.
There is a term you'll sometimes hear called "sick
building syndrome" .... I think it all started there. It
felt like a huge concrete prison to me. The only
upside to the job was that I found a way to get onto
the roof, from where you could see forever across
the Cheshire Plains and sunbathe in the summer.
My job, along with one very quiet and another very
bossy young lady, was transferring information
about customers from a piece of card onto another
piece of card. It was boring beyond belief and I
could never understand why it needed to be done
in the first place. I hated every second. I was
employed on a flexi time contract and, by the time I
finished work there, I owed them a few weeks. I
couldn't wait to get out of there as early as
possible. When they decided not to keep me on
after the 12 months, I wasn't exactly disappointed.

I decided that Doris, the Suzuki 380, was a bit
lonely, sat out there on the kerb. It was quite a
steep hill where the bike was parked and during
heavy rainstorms the street would become a
gushing torrent that would wash over the front
wheel of the bike. Doris looked very sad. Back then
I didn't even put a lock or cover on the bike. It was
quite rare for bikes to get stolen, at least compared

to today's society, where you actually expect it to happen.

I had noticed a bike for sale in the local paper and soon discovered that it was being sold by Bill Smith's Motorcycles on behalf of a private seller. I went to have a look the very next day and fell in love immediately.

I was a salesman's dream back then. I was so impulsive and impatient, that they could have sold me just about anything. However this was a nice looking bike. The fact that it was renowned for having a fragile engine with next to no power and was somewhat prehistoric in design, didn't matter. It was a 500cc bike and bigger than anything I had previously ridden.

The Honda CB500T was a twin cylinder machine and exceptionally average in every way. This was further heightened by its brown paintwork and brown seat. It radiated brownness from every nut and bolt but it's exhaust system made up for it. A Jardine 2 into 1, swept up pipe that sounded like the end of the world.... I was sold.

It was a 1976 model that was soon to be named Mabel. It was a lot of fun to ride apart from if you wanted to go any faster than 65 mph. Anything after that speed and the vibration from the old twin pot engine would make it almost impossible to keep your feet on the footpegs and required a vice like grip on the handlebars, which eventually caused your hands and arms to go completely numb. Marvellous times indeed.

As much as I loved Doris and Mabel, the need to carry a tent and associated weekend gear to distant rally venues was becoming more than just another excuse to change motorcycles.

I have no recollection who I sold Doris to, but Mabel was sold to the partner of my girlfriend's cousin, who blew the engine up a week later through a complete disregard of Mabel's delicate nature. Serves him right. Should have treated her with a lot more respect and listened to her more ...Poor old Mabel.

I had my eye on an old Honda CB750 Four F1, in Bill Smith's Motorcycle emporium.
At the time there were a number of bike shops within a not too large radius of Chester. Many a weekend would be spent visiting these halls of wonder, even if it was just to look at the same old bikes that we could never afford. Most of these places are just memories now, but Bill Smith's survived. New premises but still the same silly prices and attitude.
I went to ask about the 750 and got easily talked into spending a lot of money on a more modern Honda 750 FA, which boasted 1 more camshaft and, what Mr Honda liked to call 'Euro styling' (80's style angular design and a bit plasticky). It was very nice, quite fast, quiet and comfortable.... I didn't like it at all.
I was beginning to understand something about motorcycles.
Some bikes have character and you feel an attachment to them. They have soul and personality. They become an extension of yourself, both physically and mentally.
On the other side of this live the likes of a CB 750 FA Honda. A soulless piece of metal and plastic, with no character. Honda have managed to make this their trademark in my opinion. They don't make

bad bikes by any means, just bikes without personality. There are a few exceptions but not many.

Each to their own I say. Many people won't ride anything else and I respect that.

I never judge a fellow rider. Unless he wears one of those 'POLITE' dayglo vests to try and look like a police officer... now they're complete tossers.

In my experience, the major motorcycle manufacturers can be classified as follows …

SUZUKI..
Solid, dependable, well engineered machines with character. Probably the most consistent manufacturer of them all.

Created the underwear filling GSXR range. Ridden by fellas that don't talk much because they're on their way to the toilet.

If you owned a Katana 1100 in the 1980s you were a god.

Sportsbike fans are terrified of getting them dirty, spend half as much as the purchase price on an exhaust system and wear helmets with irridium visors.

Renowned for producing the monstrously powerful TL1000 v twin which regularly snapped frames.

Gave rebirth to the 'Hooligan' biker, with the introduction of the massively popular 'Bandit' range in 1995.

Good friends with Kawasaki.

KAWASAKI..
Fast, generally reliable, poorly finished.

Tend to be owned by clean shaven bald blokes, in their late thirties, called Dave, who wears a

'Monster' leather jacket, tight jeans and expensive trainers.

Good at making Harley Davidson clones, ridden by Harley owner clones, who have no desire to part with stupid money or spend most of their time fixing stuff.

Brought motorcycling into the modern world, with their GPZ 'R' range in the mid 80's.

If you ever uttered the words "What's that fucking racket ?" during the 1980s, it was a young lad on a Kawasaki Z650, with an Alpha 4 into 1 exhaust and a crappy mural of an album cover on the tank.

Good friends with Suzuki.

YAMAHA..

Not afraid to be different or downright nuts.

Fun bikes, some brilliant, some atrocious. Often ridiculously fast.

Made some seriously mental death machines and are solely responsible for the learner laws being changed, in the early 1980's, by introducing the World to the RD250LC.

Lead the way with the cruiser class and everyone else followed suit.

Ridden by chaps called Mike, that wear old leather jackets smelling of patchouli oil and talk too much.

Created the 'Hold on and pray' V Max, by utilising a V4 engine from one of their touring machine. An incredibly powerful bike for its time.

The R1 models are a must if you want to collect points on your licence or suffer an untimely death.

Regularly created bikes that nobody wanted for no reason at all other than they could.

HONDA..

Dependable but ultimately boring.

Keep trying to be different but not quite getting there.

Seem to specialise in making engines with poor quality chains inside, with even poorer devices to keep said chains tight.

Introduced the world to the 'Superbike', with it's CB 750 four, in 1969.

Often ridden by people called Mark, who wear their bike boots over poorly fitting jeans.

It's compulsory when a Honda rider removes his helmet to replace it with a Repsol Honda baseball cap and look around for his friends... even though he hasn't got any.

Produced the ultimate touring machine called the Goldwing, which later became a huge, soft sofa and entertainment system on wheels, that are not considered to be motorcycles at all, by anyone but their owners.

HARLEY DAVIDSON..

Overpriced toys that look cool.

Some serious enthusiasts out there but mostly middle aged, wannabe bikers.

Need to spend as much again as you paid for the bike to make it on par with their Japanese equivalents.

Usually stood next to in a carpark by men called Steve, wearing Harley branded everything, wrap around shades and bandanas.

Bike of choice for the 1%ers.

They sound nice. You can dance to the beat of a Harley... at least you can when your very, very drunk (so I've been told).

Potato, potato, potato.

BMW..

They'll take you around the globe as many times as you wish but don't try fixing anything yourself.
Usually preferred by the more sensible rider.
The GS versions are nearly always kitted out with full expedition gear, but only used for commuting or a trip to the cafe on a Sunday.
Usually ridden by men named Derek who will only talk to other BMW riders.
Ridiculously overpriced BMW riding apparel is essential, as well as helmet intercom system, so your missus can tell you to slow down.

ANYTHING ITALIAN...
Exotic and fun to ride. Garage essential or they'll become a rust machine in no time.
Need care and attention. You really have to be obsessed.
Often the choice of hipsters wearing everything retro. Brown leather jackets, a laptop case in a man bag and one of those little boot attachments that prevent the gear change lever from marking the expensive leather.
What they have plenty of is character and style, but you'll have to pay for it.
Did I mention that I love Moto Guzzis ?

TRIUMPH...
Nice bike but needs _____ (fill in the space as required).
Ridden by people who used to own the leaky versions, maniacs or blokes that want you to think they used to own the leaky versions.
Always look like they mean business, apart from the 2.3 litre Rocket 3, which looks like it's been built around a Massey Ferguson tractor engine.

Typical owner still wears a waxed cotton Belstaff jacket, or the full set of Triumph branded clothing. His name is Bob, with a fondness for Isle of Man TT Races merchandise; usually 'Busheys bar, Douglas' t-shirts and caps. Loves the smell of Castrol R.
Speed Triple versions ridden by born again nutters, that love the speed and really like to feel it.

ANYTHING FROM EASTERN EUROPE…
They are made from recycled tanks, left over from the cold war, in forced labour camps by disgruntled workers. You can tell.
Only kidding, but they are more basic than the most basic thing you can think of.
My CZ 125 would randomly seize during hot weather, but be fine after a few minutes of cooling down.

ANYTHING CHINESE...
You just don't. And just in case you do, you never will again.
There's a very good reason why brand new Chinese motorcycles are so cheap. Buy one and you'll soon find out.

Back in the room…
The weekend pilgrimages to public houses, with a place to pitch a tent went on in earnest. There were shiny rally badges to collect and it was our duty to keep the British brewery industry in business. Well somebody had to do it !
One memorable jaunt to the beautiful county of Shropshire and a lovely little pub called The

Shakespeare stands out. It was a very hot, summer weekend and the field behind the pub was full of tents and bikes.

One of the rally goers suddenly jumped on his CB900 Honda and went whizzing off, past us all, on the small road next to the camping area, only to return a few minutes later stark naked, standing with one foot on the seat of his bike, to a rapturous round of applause. It was going to be one of those weekends.

At some point during the afternoon, a crowd had gathered in front of one particular tent where a young, skinny lad was having his photograph taken, in between to young ladies. Not unusual you might think, apart from the fact that his trousers were around his ankles and the girls were holding his rather large and disproportionate penis in their hands. It was like a baby's arm holding an apple that was slowly getting bigger. It's safe to say that most of the guys attending the rally were left feeling a little inadequate. He didn't seem bothered at all.

That evening, after spending most of the afternoon drinking and feeling rather inadequate myself in the gentleman's department, I had just finished off a bottle of ginger wine and staggered across to a tent where a couple of fellas were smoking some strange smelling cigarettes. Being somewhat worse for wear, I asked to try a drag.

I don't usually smoke, never really liked it. I tried a couple of times but most of the time just ended up feeling nauseous, light headed and dizzy. I had tried a couple of puffs of cannabis before and never understood what all the fuss was about. However, on this occasion it was like somebody hit me over the head with sledgehammer. I wobbled back towards the others but didn't get very far. I could feel my stomach contents starting their escape plans and quickly made my way to the edge of the field to fertilize the local flora. I spent what seemed like an eternity puking and retching until I just fell asleep, fully clothed, draped over a barbed wire fence. I think it was a few hours until anyone noticed. It was lucky I was still wearing a leather jacket.

Due to the Honda just not doing anything for me, I advertised it in the Motorcycle News as a sale or swap. As soon as the ad appeared I was contacted by a lad with a Yamaha XV 750 Special.
During the 80's, all the major Japanese motorcycle companies created a range of 'custom' bikes. Obviously they were not customised at all but mirrored the style, with higher handlebars, shaped tanks and seats, plus lots of chrome. Yamaha referred to their models as 'US Custom' or 'Special'.
When the guy turned up to exchange the bike, he did so with a friend, who was riding pillion. Nothing unusual there, except that his friend didn't exactly have a great deal of space. The lad in front was huge. As wide as he was tall, probably around the 25 stone (160 kg) mark. Lovely bloke and over the moon about the swap. He sped away on the boring Honda with a big smile on his face. His pillion had a bit more room aswell.
This was more my style A laid back cruiser. A bit quiet for my liking and rather slow, but different. It wasn't long before I started fiddling about with it to make it more individual.
I started by adding risers to the handlebars, raising them by about 4 inches. Then I replaced the big round headlight with a pair of rectangular, halogen

spotlights, situated one above the other. I put two conical air filters onto the intake manifolds, which made the bike sound like a steam train under acceleration. Didn't make it any faster, unfortunately.

There was still something missing in my life. Then, in late 1983, during a perusal of the local newsagent, I noticed a brand new motorcycle magazine on the shelves. It was called 'Back Street Heroes.'

I had discovered a whole new religion and this was to become my bible.

CHAPTER 5

'I'm ADD and psychic. I know things ahead of time but lose track of which is which....' **Anonymous.**

One of the biggest struggles, with a wandering mind, is trying to complete any given task without breaking off to do several other tasks that spring to mind, then forgetting what it was you were doing in the first place.

My wife calls me 'Arfa', as in Arfa Job. The amount of mental effort required to see any job through to its conclusion is huge, especially if the task is mundane, like ironing for instance.

Once again, it's music that can keep me in place, at least until I'm overwhelmed by other things that I might forget about, if I don't do them *right now!*

The only way I can describe this is that it's like being surrounded by several other *'me's',* all telling me to recall, imagine or just do other things. The same other *'me's'* that over analyze every decision, scenario, situation or , well, everything that I have done or even thought about doing.

I could never be a successful criminal because I can imagine every single way that I might get caught, everything that could go wrong and every consequence of my wrongdoings.

If my wife says the slightest thing negative to me, I spiral through a thousand possible outcomes, ranging from saying nothing, to being divorced and living on the street. In fact the smallest of comments, even if obviously said in jest, can embed itself into my memory and keep getting played back, over and over again, to be worried about, dissected and questioned. Usually when I'm trying to sleep.

If I apply for a job, my mind pictures millions of different scenes, depicting another million possibilities. 'Would I be able to do the job?, what if I was useless?, will the others like me?, etc. etc.' ad nauseum ad infinitum..... like a fractal picture.

There really is no let up and people wonder why I get so tired when I appear to have done so little all day. I'm just mentally exhausted.

Amongst this constant, swirling fog lives a special type of demon.

Imagine seeing something that seriously disturbed you, an image that made you squirm and repulsed you. Now imagine being unable to switch off that image because it keeps flashing into your consciousness, relentlessly. No matter what else you try to think about, your brain is saying "Ha Ha Ha ! You're only trying to think of that to forget about THIS !" This is overwhelming because there is absolutely no escape, except to just ride it out until something else distracts you enough for your mind to let it go. But it hasn't really gone at all, it's just waiting in the wings to bother you again when there's nothing to do.

You might think that having so many ideas would be a great way to keep busy but something tags along with them.
This thing can reveal itself under many names. Impulsiveness, obsession, infatuation, impatience, to name a few.
An idea can become all consuming to the detriment of everything else. It doesn't take much once the cogs start turning and whatever it happens to be has to be done *right now*, or at least as soon as possible. My inner voices will argue against any doubts I might have and start making plans regardless of cost or consequence. These ideas can range from seeing a hill that needs running up, to life changing decisions.
I'm a lot better at controlling these impulses now, mostly due to the fact that I'm married to a

Yorkshire woman. To be quite honest, I have no idea where I'd be without her common sense, steadying influence, love and understanding. She's my anchor.

The constant need to escape the maelstrom going on in my brain makes me fidgety and restless when inactive. I pick and rub at my skin, or find something else to fiddle with (No!..not that.) in order to find some distraction through stimulation.
Even if I find something that interests me on the television, it's like trying to watch and listen with somebody knocking on every window and door, all wanting my attention. As a consequence I don't spend much time in front of the picture box unless it's a very gripping, intense and captivating film or series. Even if it is, I still fidget. Alcohol helps, unfortunately. Rubbing my wife's feet usually works best.
I find it more relaxing to play fast paced video games where I have little chance to think about anything else. My hands are busy and the voices are kept quiet. But even that gets boring after a while.
If a situation demands that I keep still and quiet, I will drum my fingers to whatever happens to be playing on my mental jukebox. If I can't do that I will grind my teeth to a tune instead.

It's a good job that I decided to join the Royal Air Force instead of the Army. I could have ended up as a sentry outside Buckingham Palace, but not for long I imagine.

As is often the case, I soon found an excuse to swap Vera, the name I had given to the Yamaha XV 750 Special. I called her that because of the V twin engine, but also because of my fondness for my Great Aunt Vera.

I loved this woman. I don't remember her being anything other than an old lady but she was just a big kid inside. I think my grandmother must have had about 50 sisters because during my childhood outings to the May Day fair in Knutsford, they seemed to be everywhere. I remember my Aunt Nancy used to sneak us kids under the fence of the fairground on Knutsford Common to avoid paying the pittance of an entry fee.

Vera was an absolute star. I recall when the floors of our house were being fixed downstairs and we were living upstairs, temporarily. Whilst looking out of the window, Vera remarked " I like it up here, you can spit on people's heads if they come to the door."

Anyway... I arranged to swap the Yamaha for a

Suzuki GS750 of unknown age and an Irish number
plate.

This was to start my love affair with 4 cylinder
Suzukis that has never really gone away.

It was painted, in a metallic, electric blue, including
the frame. It sported an Italian made 2-4 seat,
which were all the rage back then, but not that
brilliant for the pillion passenger. Best of all it had a
Yoshimura exhaust system that growled like an
angry lion and screamed like Godzilla had stepped
on a Lego brick at speed. It was just so nice to ride,
had plenty of power and could carry a fair bit of rally
equipment.

The first trip on the new steed was to the BMF
(British Motorcycle Federation) rally in
Peterborough. I think it was 1985.

The BMF were and still are, the much politer and
respectable cousins of MAG (Motorcycle Action
Group). Far too straight and sensible in my opinion
but they try. Both do a great deal to stop the
government from legislating motorcycles off the
Queens highways, but MAG were a lot more
aggressive about it.

It was a bit of a cross country trek from Chester
back then, passing through big cities on just 'A'
roads. The club had, somehow, persuaded Bill
Smith's Motorcycle Dealers to part with a fully

dressed Honda Goldwing 1200cc Aspencade for the weekend. It was the ultimate touring machine of it's time. Worth a great deal of money and as long as we advertised where it came from, we could offer people the chance to win it by throwing 6 sixes with one throw of the dice. For a small fee of course.

We had set up the stall in the knowledge that the odds of throwing 6 sixes were 46,656 to one (I just Googled it). Things were looking good. The girls had dressed in very short Evicted MCC T-shirts, that doubled as mini skirts and thigh length boots to catch the eye of prospective punters. Then the insurance company panicked and pulled out. Luckily for us the Honda UK guys were on site and were persuaded, perhaps to some degree by thigh length boots, to back us.

Apart from one heart stopping moment when one punter rolled 5 sixes, it was a huge success.

The rally sticks in the memory for two reasons. Firstly, shortly after arriving, it was time to erect the Evicted MCC flagpole. This demanded the use of a rather hefty wooden mallet to knock the pole into the ground and the expert mallet wielding abilities of Les. All went well until around the third swing of said mallet, when the hitting end decided it wasn't friends with the holding end anymore and parted company with it on the downstroke . The trajectory of the hitting end would have normally seen it making contact with the earth some feet away, leaving a large dent in the turf. That is unless somebody's genitals were not blocking it's way. Those genitals belonged to Mike. I'm pretty sure there is photographic evidence of the damage caused and I'm also pretty sure that it doesn't make for very pleasant viewing. Poor Mike.

The second reason for remembering this trip so well was getting hopelessly lost on my way home. This was a long time before sat navs and Google maps.
In my case it was a poor sense of direction and the refusal to believe that I was heading South instead of West, that led me to be a long way from where I should have been going and travelling towards London.
The problem was that I only had three quarters of a tank of fuel left, I was tired after the weekend's festivities and worst of all it was raining... a lot.
After riding for what felt like hours and actually was, I found the Motorway and realised that I still had far too many miles to go before Chester was even mentioned on the road signs. I put what change was left in my pockets towards fuel and purchased a couple of newspapers to stuff under my, already

sodden, leather jacket to provide some degree of insulation.

I was so tired by the time I reached the right Motorway junction for Chester, with still some 30 miles still to go, that I was beginning to hallucinate. I had music by the Thompson Twins playing on repeat in my head and was seeing things that couldn't possibly be there. But somehow the old Suzuki made it home.

My leather jacket weighed about the same as me and took a week to dry out. There was about a thimble full of fuel left in the tank and it took me about 2 seconds to fall asleep. All great fun.

Some refer to stuff like this as character building. Usually those that have never had to do it.

I think I remained stuck in the riding position for quite a few days following that trip. I had been on the roads, getting rained on for 8 hours solid.

Once I had recovered, the Suzuki got treated to electronic ignition, a new exhaust system and a comfy 'King and Queen' seat. Well deserved.

That bike never really let me down apart from one of the exhaust downpipes falling off on the M5, coming home from a rally near Worcester. The engine note suddenly changed and I caught a glimpse of the wayward exhaust header disappearing under the wheels of a truck.

The Suzuki GS model engines were very much over-engineered and ultra reliable. The electrical system didn't like wet weather much and the brakes required a fair amount of effort on the riders behalf to bring the whole thing to stop at anything over 40 mph. But great bikes.

I have owned a Suzuki GS250, 550, 650, 750 and 2 GS 850s. Also a GSX750 which boasted twice as many engine valves... mine also had luminous pink wheels as mentioned previously.

I accidentally roasted a sparrow between the exhaust pipes of that bike. It was a very early morning trip (5am) to a rally in North Wales and involved dodging suicidal local wildlife of every description. The sparrow was not so lucky.

Having a high speed minds pays dividends when riding. It can take in huge amounts of information and prepares you for things that might happen, so there is little in the way of unexpected events. It allows you to use things while negotiating traffic that most people will never think of, such as using house and shop windows to see reflections of vehicles around bends and corners. Birds flying from hedges and trees as approaching, unseen cars or bikes drive past. Moving windscreen wipers and lights on approaching vehicles, to let you know that there's nasty weather ahead. Then there's the knowledge that people carriers often contain screaming kids and distracted drivers... to name but a few.

However, as my old Ninjitsu teacher used to say... "There is no defence against a sucker punch."

As much as I loved the Suzuki, there was still this need, fuelled by newly found bible, 'Back Street Heroes' magazine, to build the ultimate chopper. I had the donor bike in mind; The Yamaha XS650 twin.

Built by Mr Yamaha as a direct assault on Triumph's market leading T140 Bonneville, It had the classic looks, reliability, simplicity and relative affordability, that made it a favourite amongst custom bike builders. At least those who couldn't afford a Harley Davidson.

The Suzuki got traded in, at Wrexham Scooters, for a standard model Yamaha, which turned out to be as inspiring to ride as an old donkey with haemoroids on Blackpool beach. However, I had big plans for her .... huge in fact. I wanted every modification possible, that was considered 'de rigueur ' at the time.

The frame was to be hardtailed (No suspension)

and goose necked (stretched at the front). It was to have 12 inch over length forks. It had to have a 2 and a half gallon mustang petrol tank. The yolks, which held the forks in place, were to be widened, which meant spacers had to be made for the brake discs. The rear wheel would be rebuilt to make it a wider 16 inch version. It needed a single, sprung seat, a mini speedometer and a multitude of shiney bits from various catalogues and my hyperactive imagination. Then there was the paint.

From the outset this was going to be a disaster. The best way is to keep things simple and this went way beyond simplicity, common sense and a realistic budget. I wanted a show winning bike but would eventually be left with an almost unrideable pile of junk.

I stripped everything down with little thought about how it would all go back together.

I sent the frame off to be modified and it came back with the front part being extended by the use of different diameter tubing. It looked a mess.

I enlisted the skills of a supposed engineer, who advertised in Back Street Heroes, to make some wide yokes and disc spacers. This engineer turned out to be alcoholic old hippy who had convinced himself that he knew how to create finely and precisely engineered pieces of motorcycle artistry, when in fact they were just badly machined lumps of cheap steel that only looked the part. I should have been worried when he insisted on sampling some of my unfinished home brew beer, many weeks before it was ready. I imagine he's dead by now.

I ordered the extended forks without even thinking about how to compensate for the length of springs inside them, or how I was going to extend the speedometer cable, which ran off the front wheel. Let alone where I was going to find a brake hose that was 12 inches longer.

I then realised that I had nowhere to mount my handlebars, speedo or something to stop the yokes from turning too far and hitting my nice new mustang tank.

Things got even better when I had the rear wheel rebuilt with a nice new 16 inch alloy rim and stainless steel spokes. It looked fantastic until I took it to have nice new chunky Avon tyre fitted, only to be told that there was no hole in the rim for the tyre valve to go through.

Then there was the paint....

I had eventually decided on a dark green paint scheme with a very subtle finish of ivy leaves coming down the side of the tank, with the words 'Sweet Leaf' on the top of the tank. The name of a Black Sabbath song about marijuana as it happens.

Once again I contacted another supposed expert from the pages of my glossy bible and he came to collect my frame and tank.

After what seemed to be forever, mainly because it was, they were returned. I know I asked for subtle leaves, but there's subtle and there's almost invisible, it was crap. Things were not going well at all.

I was not to be defeated though. I had some success when I had some forward controls made by Crazy Odge, who had recently started another, and far better, custom bike/lifestyle magazine called 'AWOL'. It was a much more realistic view of the biker scene, with bikes that hadn't cost a fortune to create and had been built by blokes in sheds with limited resources but a lot more ability than me.

I slowly pieced everything back together, discovering more and more things I hadn't thought about along the way, until it was ready for it's first ride.

It was more of a tentative wobble in reality, but I was sure it looked cool. One thing for sure, It was bloody loud.

It needed an MOT, so I steadily rode it to an old school mate's, fathers garage near Chester. He was on his dinner break when I arrived but I instantly knew of his return by the shouts of "Get that piece of shit out of my garage ! I'm not MOTing that thing."

I can't actually remember who passed it, but they must have been a bit lacking in grey matter, drunk, or had lost their glasses.

It was a complete pig to ride. The seat was uncomfortable and far too bouncy, it handled like an overloaded shopping trolley with a broken wheel and the brakes were like something off a clown's bike from the circus.

I ended up putting it up for a swap as an ongoing project and was shortly in possession of a Suzuki GS650 Katana. A strangely styled rocket ship in silver, orange and black. The best thing about it was that it was rideable. I liked it a lot. For a while at least.

Styled in true 80's garishness, it was great fun to ride and had a power band like a 2 stroke. Mine had no ignition key and a 4 inch long 'silencer' that did everything but silence. To get it started I had to twist two wires together and hope for the best. Those were the days.

I am very aware, whilst writing this, that the timeline has not been completely linear and there are many gaps and inconsistencies in my recollections (with some poor grammar to boot), but this reflects my life at the time.

I was completely taken over by the need to create and the need to be a responsible adult with a job, bills to pay and a roof to keep over my head.

I was, until very recently, completely useless with money. I just couldn't keep track of what I had to spend and on what. The most important thing was always whatever was occupying my mind at the time to the detriment of everything else.

I was working the night shift at the Royal Mail in Chester whilst living in Buckley, some 13 miles away. I would make this journey on my bike regardless of whether it was summer or winter, with a good helping of snow and temperatures well below freezing. I had no other choice. There were many times when, finishing a shift, that I would get to my bike, only to find that the sponge filling of the seat, which tended to hold water, as sponges tend to do, would be frozen into a solid block of ice. Nice.

I recall one trip back home, following a 12 hour shift. I was riding my partners Suzuki TS 100 trials bike. I remember leaving work, then, the next thing I knew I woke up about 200 yards from my house at the crossroads in Buckley. Seeing a red traffic light in front of me, I grabbed the brakes and proceeded to fall off, in what would have been a very embarrassing incident. Luckily everyone was still tucked up in bed and missed the entertainment.

One hurt knee and a bent brake lever were the only casualties.

What was slowly creeping up on me was depression.
The whole being a responsible adult thing was getting on top of me. I started to retreat back into myself, make myself ill and start wondering if it was all worth while. I wasn't eating or sleeping properly and was looking pale and gaunt.
The truth of the matter is that I had absolutely no idea what I was doing anymore and simply didn't care. The worst thing about it was that nobody else seemed to be bothered either. I was in a relationship but felt lonely and hopeless.
Maybe a few kind words, or a bit of support would have pulled me out of that big black hole. It just never happened.

The demons had seen their chance and were coming out to play.

CHAPTER 6

'Sensitive people usually love deeply and hate deeply. They don't know any other way to live than by extremes because their emotional thermostat is broken.'
— **Shannon L. Alder**

The trouble with suppressing so many thoughts, feelings, emotions, etc. Is that there is a pressure cooker effect. Sometimes I can feel it building inside me like a volcano preparing to erupt. Fortunately this is very rare and I have some coping mechanisms, which usually involves me becoming withdrawn and distant, often for a few days. This gets mistaken for being upset, being in a bad mood or that something is wrong. This is not the case, It's just my way of calming the mind and letting things go.

I will often meditate and let everything come to the surface of my mind and let thoughts drift away. However there are some extremely rare times when another side of me will show itself.

I am a very peaceful, calm and quiet person but if my family, friends or property are threatened, the lid blows off the pressure cooker and I lose all sense of fear, danger or consequence. I scare myself at times.

When I was younger and fitter, this release came through sports. I was not particularly strong or skilled but made up for it with sheer aggression. Much to the dismay of my PE teachers, the pale, skinny kid, that was always picked last for team games, would outrun and fearlessly tackle anyone on a rugby pitch regardless of their size.

The concentrated mass of tension would get released and I became a blur on the running track or long jump. Never judge a book by it's cover they say.

During my short stay in the Royal Air Force I was picked to train for their hurdles team. I doubt anyone would have bet on that ever happening a few years earlier.

In more recent times, I found a release through snowboarding. It requires a great deal of concentration and is often bloody terrifying. Apart from the physical side of snowboarding, there's the absolute peace, beauty and sheer grandeur of the mountains, which is enough of a distraction on their own. I always feel at peace amongst the snow covered peaks.

Keeping things bottled up, overthinking everything

and stacking scenarios has a very detrimental effect on self esteem. Imagining every scenario creates worries about how people see you and becoming introverted is the escape mechanism.

I am a very quiet person because I convince myself that nobody is interested in anything I have to say. I have visualised every meeting and conversation a thousand times, each a different version, so I am already bored with it myself before I speak. So I imagine it to be just as boring to everyone else.

I find it far easier to express myself with written words and have recently started writing poetry and a novel, which is incredibly therapeutic.

This lack of confidence reveals itself in other ways. Being over sensitive to criticism, getting overemotional and lacking tolerance are just a few. On the other hand such depths of thought enable a great deal of empathy for others with similar problems.

Trying to be all things to all people is a constantly shifting state, yet seeing everything from every possible angle enables me to become a social chameleon. I am able to completely change my character and approach to any situation. It is One of the many advantages of this condition.

I often think I should have been on the stage. I have recently discovered that a great many of my

favourite actors also have ADHD, Anthony Hopkins
and Keanu Reeves for instance. This came as no
surprise whatsoever because they must have a
huge depth of imagined experience to work with
and be able to rehearse inside their minds.

You see, it really isn't all bad news. You can wallow
in self pity or make the most of what life has given
you.

To quote Lewis Carroll's Cheshire Cat, from Alice in
Wonderland, " I'm not crazy, my reality is just
different from yours".

I have the Cheshire Cat tattooed on the back of my
right hand as a constant reminder.

The endless flow of images, sounds, ideas and
words brings about creativity. I can draw pictures
that my mind creates and write songs and poems
from a single word popping into my head, while my
brain provides me with the rest.

I can change and become a character in my book
in an instant, because I have imagined being that
other person many times. Nothing shocks or
surprises me because I've played every scenario to
every possible event on a constant, evolving loop. I
have no real plan when I write fiction. The story just
grows and evolves as I'm writing, taking on a life of
its own. It often feels like there's somebody else
doing it for me.

I can see things around me that most people never take the time to look at. I question everything and take nothing for granted. I feel energy and *'see'* words. I can visualise anything in minute detail and compose music in my mind.

I can hold conversations with myself and imagine things that are beyond reality. I can see through the surface and find beauty in people and things that are often overlooked.

The best thing is, I am never bored... ever.

The secret is to embrace what I have and adapt accordingly.

I have been prescribed various medications, but all they did was change who I was. It was OK at first, but I found that I was viewing myself from the perspective of another person and what I saw was nothing like me at all.

All that medication did for me was to give me an energy boost in the morning only to slam me to the ground by the afternoon. It took away a part of me that I had become friends with, that had grown with me and I considered totally normal. It left me feeling empty and cold.

The creativity ceased and was replaced by overconfidence and cheekiness that I never used to possess. I started feeling aggressive and began to have some really bad thoughts, which was never the case before my meds.

I finally realised, that although I knew what the problem was, that it wasn't really a problem at all. It was just how I was meant to be.

The relief when I stopped taking this medicine was like coming home to a nice warm duvet. Finding comfort in the familiar.

Back in the 1980s , I was totally unaware of these things. Life had become a blur of debts, problems and confusion. I was making myself sick with worry but didn't know how to make things right. I was working 12 hour nights and any weekend work I could get, but getting nowhere. I was becoming a ghost.

I could see it in many of my co-workers but never imagined that I would become the same as them. Living beyond their means, via lots of overtime and just existing. Yet that is exactly what I was doing. No time to live, just work, work, work and nothing to show for it all.

I would often find myself riding home, in the early hours of the morning, on the empty dual carriageway towards North Wales, with voices in my head saying, '*What if you were to just open up that throttle and close your eyes?... you won't feel a thing and you'll finally have a bit of peace.*' I simply

didn't care anymore. Life meant absolutely nothing
and the light at the end of tunnel had snuffed itself
out.

I had drifted apart from the Evicted club, not
through any bad feeling, they were (and still are)
great people. It was mainly due to my state of mind
and the depression into which I was slowly sinking.
Because I was consumed by the building of my 650
chopper, there was a space which needed to be
filled, in order for me to get to work, if nothing else.
I received a phone call from Dugdales Motorcycles
to let me know about a bike they had just taken in
part exchange that I might be interested in. I can't
remember how they knew I wanted a cheap bike,
but somehow they did. A great deal that happened
during those years is lost inside a big dark cloud.

The bike was a Yamaha SR500. They had been
producing a 500cc single cylinder off road bike,
known as the XT500, for many years and decided
that the engine might work in a standard road
chassis. It did, to a point.
Bits used to fall off when least expected to, due to
the vibration of the engine. When left on it's centre
stand it would perform a complete 360 degree
rotation for the same reason. It could only be
started by means of a kick start that required a

great deal of skill and timing to avoid it kicking back and breaking your leg, which it attempted to do on several occasions. It was remarkably slow, didnt handle particularly well and held all of its engine oil inside the frame. Despite all of this I really liked it. It was different, great fun to ride and quirky; Things that have always appealed to me.

The vibration caused no end of problems including working loose the nuts which adjusted the tappets, leaving them rattling around the top of the engine. Not a good thing. Luckily they were easy to get at and fix.

I just loved the feel of the single cylinder engine. It felt like I was actually riding something, if that makes sense? It was raw and basic, nasty and dirty, weird and wonderful.

It finally repaid my love for it by self destructing on the way home from work at 6am in the middle of nowhere. An engine valve got stuck and the big piston came up to greet it, in a catastrophic sort of meeting. Thanks for that, Mr Fully Synthetic Oil.

I sold it for parts to an old schoolmate who shared my love of living with a problem motorcycle.

I had been invited by a club from Connahs Quay, called the Hare and Hounds MCC, who met in a pub of the same name. A bit of a rowdy, ragtag bunch of old school bikers but good people. It was only a short ride away so I knew the SR500 would make it without losing too many important parts. It was being held at a roadside pub in the countryside, just outside Mold, in an idyllic spot know as Loggerheads.

We were all outside, in the pub car park, when we heard the distant rumble of approaching bikes. Two heavily customised bikes swung into the car park at speed. One of them was an old British bike with massively extended forks that cut through the crowd, scattering the hordes of happy drinkers. A very scruffy, unkempt guy with long black hair and a big black beard staggered off the bike. The 'Henchmen MC' had arrived.

These guys had a fearsome reputation in that part of North Wales, but have since become part of a much bigger club.

After downing a beer he placed the empty bottle on the floor, in the middle of the crowded car park and attempted to refill it using his own bodily fluids. This was made all the more difficult by the fact that he was already rather unsteady and more than a little under the influence. Despite their grand entrance, everyone just carried on enjoying the summer sun. Nothing much phases a bunch of bikers.

I still know the bloke with the poor aim. He shall remain nameless but he's alright, even after all these years. Some people just seem to be indestructible.

I don't think I was very popular in the small cul de sac where I lived in Buckley. To be honest I didn't really like it there either.

To be fair to the neighbours, the driveway was usually populated by various motorcycles, in different states of repair or customisation and there was a regular flow of visiting 'undesirables' on strange looking and rather loud machinery.

At some point a local resident and self appointed spokesman for everyone that he had probably never even spoken to, decided to walk across the road to complain about the 'mess' on my driveway. I politely suggested that he take himself and his opinions back across the road and refrain from even thinking about stepping foot on my property ever again (perhaps in a slightly less polite manner). It wasn't even that bad.

A few days later he dropped dead.... Nothing to do with me I hasten to add. Funnily enough there was never another word mentioned about the bikes or the, so called, 'mess'.

The only plus side to living in Buckley was the Tivoli night club, which hosted quite a few famous rock bands of the time, and it was only a short walk away.

It's still going to this day and still has rock bands playing there. It's a bit of a dump to be honest and hasn't changed that much since the 1980s, but nobody seems to care. Rock fans aren't interested in how a place looks, just the music.

Bands such as Dr Feelgood, The Quireboys and Love Hate played there and often just joined the crowd for a drink after the gig. Great days.

But I digress, again.

For some inexplicable reason an ad in the local paper caught my eye. It was for a bike and sidecar combination. I suddenly had visions of riding this contraption with a dog in the sidecar and loads of room to carry luggage. My impulsive nature took complete control and shortly afterwards I was a few hundred quid worse off and trying to figure a way to get a, non running, Jawa 350 combination back home from 20 miles away. Can't remember how that happened but it soon joined the family of bikes on the overcrowded, oil stained driveway.

If you want a basic bike then you won't find anything more basic than a Jawa (except perhaps an MZ). They hail from what used to be know as Czechoslovakia and I believe the were assembled in a factory full of mentally retarded political prisoners with a real grudge against the Western side of Europe. They were given big hammers and instructions in Swahili to create something out of scrap metal, to be sold to people who couldn't believe how cheap they were. There's a reason why, believe me.

Only kidding. I don't know how they're made, but the are about as basic as it's possible to get. Everything on the bike is functional and nothing more.

The first job was to get the old twin cylinder engine running. Eventually, with the assistance of a friend, it fired into life in a puff of blue smoke and the familiar 'ding da ding ding' of an ancient 2 stroke motor. Things were looking good. I wheeled the whole thing onto the road, pulled in the clutch, engaged first gear, slowly released the clutch and went rapidly backwards ! That wasn't supposed to happen. I'm pretty sure a little bit of wee sneaked out.

I never really got the hang of having something bolted to the side of a bike. If you accelerated the bike would try to go around the sidecar and if you braked, the sidecar would try to come around the bike. Nope... not for me. I eventually sold the sidecar for as much as I had bought the whole combination for and left the bike outside until the gypsies pinched it. They were welcome to it.

More out of boredom than anything else, I decided to try and start my own club, known as 'Lowriders Nationwide.'
The idea was to create a non-commital club for people that were into custom motorcycles.
I put an ad in Back Street Heroes and got a few responses and met some great people. I even had some t-shirts printed, that were really quite cool.
Unfortunately, following a particularly suspect visit and a much more obvious letter, from a local 1% club, I decided it would be a lot easier to just forget the whole idea.
It was an innocent attempt to create something different, but the biker's world is often a very peculiar animal indeed. You have to learn how to tread very carefully.

It would appear like I was having a great time back then but the reality was quite another thing. The monotony of everyday life was dragging me down. In an attempt to change things for the better, I decided to sell the house. What I didn't expect to happen was for it to be sold within a few hours of it going up in the estate agent's window.

It was time to move fast and find somewhere else to live.

The move back to my birth town of Chester didn't really help a great deal. The new house was in an area called Blacon. The full name of which was Blacon Cum Crabwall, which makes it sounds rather upper class and respectable. It isn't.
Blacon is one of the biggest council estates in Europe. There are a few nice parts of it but on the whole it is populated by people on low incomes or benefits and more than its fair share of criminals and lowlifes, who will do just about anything to get their next fix.
There are good people too of course, plenty of them, but everybody who chooses to live there does so in the full knowledge that they will have to deal with more than their fair share of trouble. I have spent many years there so know this to be true.
On one occasion I had a motorcycle stolen when I parked it in the City Centre, on a lunch break from work. The police called me to say they had found my bike in a field near Blacon... surprise, surprise. When I arrived there to collect it, they had a group of young lads in custody, one of which was the son of my next door neighbour. That just about tells you all you need to know about the place.

I started selling, buying and swapping bikes again, just to try and add some excitement to my life. It was during this time I discovered Moto Guzzis. Pronounced 'Motto Gootsi', they are Italian motorcycles produced in Lombardy and are the oldest, continuous producer of motorcycles in Europe. I instantly fell in love with my new bike. Although I am A Cancerian and fall in love very easily.

My newly acquired, but heavily used and abused, machine was a SP1000 Spada. Guzzi's touring model of the time, with hard luggage and a two part fairing to keep the British weather at bay. What I discovered was just how well the bike handled. I could throw it through any bend with more confidence than ever. It would just glue itself to the road and change direction as easily as me just thinking about it. I would often scare people who were riding behind me, due the how far I could lean the Moto Guzzi over when negotiating bends. It felt like nothing to me.

I loved the grunt of the 90 degree v twin engine too. Instant torque and power. Not the fastest thing in the World but it just felt so good.

I believe this is where my fondness for big, twin cylinder bikes originated from.

I always regretted selling that bike and have no real idea why I did. Another reason lost in the whirlwind of my mind. I have always liked the idea of another Moto Guzzi but the lack of a garage has always stopped me. They don't take too kindly to being left outside in the British climate.

I think I was still looking for ways to distract my racing brain and kick myself out of the ever deepening hole of depression. In reality, I was just making things worse.
On a random visit to Dugdale's, I spotted the possible answer.
Sat on display was a, nearly new, Kawasaki GPZ900R. This was the ultimate bike of it's time and I was probably drooling on the floor. I couldn't really afford it but I had to have it... right now !
Finance agreement signed and a long week's wait followed.
When the day finally arrived, what seemed like months later, I nervously made my way to the dealers. I had never owned a bike so new or modern. I didn't know what to expect but my stomach was doing cartwheels in anticipation. The gleaming beast was sat there waiting for me, resplendent in silver, red and black. I tentatively swung my, slightly trembling, leg over the seat and lifted the bike off it's side stand. Turning the key

and pressing the start button, started the engine purring beneath me. I clicked the gearbox into first gear and steadily made my way off the forecourt and onto the country road.

Now you must understand that I had been riding bikes from a different era before this sparkling new monster. They were a lot less powerful than the GPZ and had brakes that only worked if you really gripped the lever. The power was easy to get used to, just a little more delicate use of clutch on throttle. I gently and smoothly coasted onto the tarmac and decided I was gathering speed a little too quickly, as the road was on a gradient, so I grabbed the front brake lever as I had been used to. The bike stopped... dead on the spot. After dangling in mid air for a split second, I just managed to put my feet down before the whole thing crashed to terra firma. Phew ! Note to self, 'The brakes work rather well. Only one finger required.'

On the bypass I decided to open up the throttle a little, just to see how well it responded. Most of my bikes had struggled to reach 100 mph before now, so imagine my surprise when looking down at the speedo to see and indicated 125 mph with little or no effort on the bikes behalf. Of course the speedo must have been faulty because I would never go that fast on a 70mph public road. Obviously.

This was a whole new World to me. It was a dream to ride, apart from a very twitchy 16 inch front wheel and carburettors that iced up regularly. But as per usual after a few months, I began to find it all to clinical, too plastic and far too 'nice'. It was much too clean and shiny to use for commuting when there was salt on the roads and I had to rinse it down with cold water every time I got home from work.

I eventually sold it and paid off the finance company after just a few months.

I didn't know what I wanted anymore, not just with motorcycles, with my whole life. It felt like I was living in an alien World where everyone else seemed happy and content with the universe. I was nothing like them.

I had this intense, burning energy, clawing away inside my skull. Nothing was satisfying my restlessness or letting my mind rest. If I had known that this was a mental health problem then maybe I could have done something about it, but I didn't and the truth is, nobody did. The trouble was that I couldn't even explain it to anyone and, apart from anything else, I was feeling desperately lonely, despite the fact that I was married.

This darkness creeping over me manifested itself through my next motorcycle.

Desperate not to be without 2 wheel transport, I bought an imported Honda CB750 FA. I didn't really like them but it was very cheap and fulfilled a purpose. It was in quite good condition overall, then one day I just looked at and had a vision. Just a few hours later it was transformed into 'BABYLON'.

I had cut away the rear subframe to make it a single seater, mounted the rear light and number plate on the, now redundant, rear footpeg mounts, made a seat out of my old leather jacket, sprayed everything satin black and painted the word Babylon on each side of the tank, in big white letters. I bought an old, slightly ratty, Harris exhaust system off EBay. It finished the whole thing off perfectly and had this wonderful effect when you opened the throttle. There would be a short pause, as if the exhaust was quietly collecting all the noise and power from the engine, then it would spit it all out of the end can in a symphony of raucous sound. The bike looked mean as fuck. It was dark, moody and aggressive. Everything I was feeling at the time had been transformed into that piece of Japanese metal. I rode it that way too.

One of my work colleagues was so impressed with how it looked, he offered me a small fortune to

125

persuade me to part company with the beast. I
resisted for a while but he eventually wore me
down. It was double what I had paid for it.
That was a bad move. It took away something I had
created out of my feelings, thoughts and
personality. It was the outlet for the twisting,
writhing demon trapped inside me. It should have
told me right away that I needed help but I didn't
listen.

By now I was barely clinging onto my last strands of
sanity. I was careless, thoughtless and hopeless. I
was living in a huge black hole, devoid of feelings
and with a selfish disregard for anybody or
anything. It felt like I was completely alone and that
nobody could give a shit whether I lived or died.

Something had to give.

CHAPTER 7

'Maybe we all have darkness inside of us and some of us are better at dealing with it than others.'
— **Jasmine Warga, My Heart and Other Black Holes**

The hyperactive part of my condition is all in the brain, but decided to reveal itself a little more during puberty.

I didn't realise it at the time, but on reflection, if I had been my parents, I would have been tempted to have my head examined by the men in white coats. Then again, they didn't take much notice of anything I was doing.

I would pull stupid faces and strut around talking nonsense, in a posh accent, like I was a narrator for Pathe News in the 1940s. I was out of control, not naughty, just downright stupid. I think the only member of my family to notice my strange behaviour was my brother, when he came home on leave from the Army.

There was very little to do at home and I had no friends living close by, so had to find my own entertainment. I tried my hand at various different hobbies but didn't have the focus or concentration to persevere with any of them.

There was an old upright piano in the house and, for some strange reason. I had chosen music as one of my options to study during my final two terms at school. What possessed me to do this I have no idea. I think it must have been the lesser of several evils.

I couldn't read music because, like algebra, my brain simply refused to make sense of it.

I couldn't play the piano at all, even though I attended quite a few lessons, but anything I was taught refused to stay in my head and flew away like loose notes of paper in the wind, with the words, 'Not important', written on them.

I had to drag myself into Chester, on the bus, to sit with a very strange woman and attempt to convert little dots and symbols into finger movements on a keyboard. I just couldn't.

When it came to my music exam, I was plonked in front of a piano, given some sheet music and asked to play the tune. I sat there, sweating profusely, and managed to play just a single note. At least it was the right one… C, if I recall correctly.

With nothing else to do, I would often get on my pushbike and ride for miles, on the busy A41 out of Chester, to Beeston Castle. I would hide the bike in the bushes, strip off and run around the Cheshire countryside naked. I needed to burn off the hissing pressure cooker of mental energy, but it just wouldn't stop.

I was like a squirrel on amphetamine. Everything seemed to be rushing madly around me in a blur. It felt like I was trapped on a rock, surrounded by the raging torrent of a river in full flood. The worst thing was that I wasn't able to tell anyone about it.

Apart from my newly found fondness for masturbation, there was no release for all of this inner tension. That did help a little... must be said.

I don't know what it is about getting naked, perhaps it's a form of escape from the drudgery and burdens of modern life. All I know is that it felt good. Plus there was the added danger of getting caught. My old bedroom window opened onto a sloped kitchen roof. I would strip off and climb out there on summer nights, just lying there looking up at the stars in the cool night air.

Perhaps it's a family trait. My sister is an avid naturist and spends most of her time naked. I imagine living in a warm climate helps with that. Sunshine has an aphrodisiac effect on me, so nudist beaches would probably result in me refusing to come out of the sea or lying on my stomach all the time.

I don't need much persuasion to start frolicking through the countryside in my birthday suit, nettles permitting. I just feel sorry for anyone that sees me doing it. I hear therapy is quite expensive.

The school expected me to make decisions regarding my future during this hormone fuelled and confusing time.

I hadn't got a clue what was happening in the present, so how the hell could I decide what I wanted to do in the future?

I was so distracted by the electrical storm going on behind my eyes, I nearly got flattened by an articulated wagon when I was riding home from school. I just rode out of a side road, straight into it's path. My brain simply didn't see him through the mental fog. The driver was not even slightly amused but thankfully wide awake. My mind was

spinning out of control and I was finding it difficult to
do anything right.

I would often do daft things, in the middle of the
night, mostly because sleep was the last thing my
brain ever had in mind.
Sometimes I would creep out of the window, down
the roof and climb over the wall into next door's
garden. For no other reason than the adrenaline
rush of doing something wrong.

Waking up at some unearthly hour, thoughts arrive
like raindrops on a still pond. They create ripples
until more raindrops fall and the ripples cross each
other, forming a swirling pattern with no order or
form. A quantum mess of ever-changing pictures,
shapes and sound. A torrential downpour of
nonsense. Sleep deserts me.
It's not like I'm consciously thinking about anything
but my brain demands that I do. It assaults me with
random thoughts like they're written on a cricket bat
and I'm hit in the face with it. Unless I'm very, very
tired, that's it .... I'm awake.
It happened this very morning (not the 'creeping
into next door's garden' bit by the way).

My eyes flickered open to see the bright red LEDs indicating 0115. The little internal switch clicked to the on position and the next thing I knew I was thinking about this very chapter. It was like fireworks going off inside my head. One thought at a time would have been nice, but that's just not how it works for me.

This is a common scenario for me I'm afraid. 'Early hours inspiration' I call it.

In the latter part of the 1980s I found a new way to focus my mind.

Music has been a constant companion for me. It is in my head at all times and as soon as I wake up in the morning there is something playing on my mental jukebox.

The strange thing is that, perhaps because of the way my grey matter perceives things, I 'see' music. It is never just sound, but a constant collage of pictures, colours and shapes. Always moving, as if I'm travelling through a tunnel, not unlike an arty music video.

I not only see it, but feel it too. It can wrap me in a warm blanket, give me goose bumps, or punch me in the stomach. It all depends on what comes through those headphones or jumps out of the speakers. I wouldn't have it any other way.

I feel the energy of live music so strongly that it can move me to tears. If I hear a song that I grew up listening to, performed by the original artist, emotions swell up inside me and burst out of my eyes. Can't help it and I ain't ashamed to admit it.

Chester had a lot of rock fans with nowhere to go, so along with my friend and cousin of my wife at the time, Pete, (known to us at the time as 'Zeppo', a shortened version of Zeppelin Belly, for obvious reasons.) we decided that we could fill that void.
I had a huge record collection on vinyl and between us, we cobbled together a DJ mixing desk, a few lights and a couple of big speakers.
A willing venue was discovered, within walking distance of the city centre, called the South View Community Centre, which today is buried beneath some very expensive, waterside apartments.
The first night went down rather well. We had no idea whether the built in amplifier of the record decks would be powerful enough to fill the space with sound, so we hired a 1000 watt slave amp. We needn't have worried. We had the volume set between zero and one and it was still bloody loud.
We had planted the seeds and word soon got around.
The second week saw the place full to bursting.
The centre decided not to charge us a fee for hiring

the place, due to the huge amount of money they took behind the bar. They did have to order a lot more cases of Newcastle Brown Ale however. Zeppo became more of a silent partner to be honest. He had the uncanny ability to completely empty a dance floor.

One of the biggest mistakes a fledgling DJ makes is playing only the songs that they like. It simply doesn't work that way. You have to read the crowd and think like they do. A big clue was the way they dressed and which bands were displayed on their t-shirts. Easy really.

For some reason Zeppo seemed to think that the whole thing made him some sort of celebrity come rock star. We really were not at all. I just loved playing the music loud and watching the crowd enjoy themselves. I enjoy sharing the things I love with others and, to me at least, that was payment enough.

I loved the concentration needed to keep the punters dancing and happy. The tracks needed choosing and planning a few tunes into the future. Then they had to be cued up and started at exactly the right time, to mix perfectly with the last track ending. One faded in while the other is faded out. It required an expert knowledge of exactly how songs started and finished. Very satisfying when it was

done just right. Nowadays it's all done for you, bar
the choice of music.

The worst part of it back then was humping around
big crates of LPs and singles, along with a massive
mixing turntable, speakers, lights and cables. Good
fun though. It can all be done with a couple of
speakers, an amplifier and a smart phone
nowadays. Much easier.

We started booking local bands to play at the
centre with a great deal of success. To such a
degree that we had to employ security in the form
of a doorman named 'Mouse'. A very quiet and
respectful guy unless you gave him a good reason
to be otherwise.

On one such occasion he escorted a young guy out
of the building because he was being aggressive
towards his own girlfriend. A few minutes later he re
entered the centre with a view to causing trouble,
but immediately came face to face with Mouse's fist
and exited the door backwards. He thought better
about trying it a second time.

We called ourselves the 'Crazy Train Rock Disco'
after Ozzy Osbourne's hit song and finished every
night with that track.

It was at the height of a glam rock resurgence, due
to bands like Motley Crue, Faster Pussycat and
Guns'n'Roses, so I dressed the part. Hair right
down my back, stretch jeans, cowboy boots in

stitched brown leather with brass toe caps, an 'L.A. Guns' t-shirt under a mint green, pinstripe jacket, with various dangly bits attached to parts of my clothing and anatomy. I drew the line at make up, but I did get my hair permed a couple of times.

A few characters stand out in the memory from those nights. There was Scott, who used to just run around the outside of the dance floor like a lunatic and Ozzy, a huge young lad with an Ozzy Osbourne tattoo, who used to carry Scott on his shoulders when an ACDC track was played. They were a fantastic bunch and never gave us a spot of bother. Just a constant barrage of requests.

At one point the self, imagined, rock star status of Zeppo went to his head and he decided to try and venture into the big time promotions business, by booking the band 'Gwar' to play at a large venue in Wrexham. I knew this was a step too big for us to take and told him to go it alone. My cautiousness was rewarded when the band found out that he was a complete nobody and backed out at the last minute. leaving him with a venue to fill and a lot of pissed off Gwar fans to appease or refund. I must admit to having a quiet little smirk to myself about that one.

Zeppo never did become a celebrity or rock star. I believe he's somewhere up in the executive ranks

of the Royal Mail nowadays. Best of luck to him.
I don't recall why those rock nights came to an end,
but big changes in my life were on the horizon and
looming larger with each day.

I sold the Moto Guzzi for the usual reasons. This
just left me with no bike and consequently a great
big void in, my already very gloomy, existence. I
tried changing my shift pattern at the Royal Mail,
but I was still caught up in the work, eat, sleep,
repeat cycle. An unstimulated ADD/ADHD fuelled
brain can only tolerate that for so long. I ended up
back on 12 hour night shifts again, amongst the
postal ghosts. Things just went from bad to worse.

Whether it has something to do with ADHD I don't
know, but whenever I'm with someone I like to pay
them a lot of attention and show a lot of affection.
When this is not a reciprocal, I become confused
and eventually paranoid. The cogs start spinning
and the tiniest worry or doubt gets magnified and
dwelled upon until it becomes all consuming. Some
call it being over sensitive, maybe It is. All I know is
that I can't help it.
In my already depressed state, the slightest
negative word or action would be felt as a hammer
blow to my heart. On the other side of the scale,

the slightest show of kindness or affection would have me nearly in tears.

The darkness had got hold of me and there was just a faint glimmer of light in the distance, so I walked towards that light leaving every single part of my old life behind to start a new one. But that's another story.

Fast forward to the 21st century.....

Trying to be all things to all people had left me deeply hurt and losing sight of who I really was. I needed to find myself again.

I had brought myself to the conclusion, that no matter what I tried to do, or who I tried to be, it would never be good enough.

I am a naturally chilled out, easy going person, with a mind as open as the ocean itself. I treat people with kindness and compassion. I'm neither aggressive or forceful. I have many faults, as we all do, but try to be the best person that I can be for everyone in my life. Unfortunately this has often left me open to having my good nature taken advantage of and seriously abused. Despite having more than my fair share of tolerance, I have it stretched to it's limit at times. My lip has the bite marks to prove it.

To put it in simple terms, some people have treated
me like shit.

More out of boredom than anything else, I decided
to enlist the services of the World Wide Web.
I had heard about internet dating, but had become
a little too cynical to be that bothered with it all. I
had given up on ever finding 'The One'. They
simply didn't exist.
Regardless of this, I posted a daft picture of myself
with a snowboard, taken somewhere in the French
Alps and a short bio, on a free website.
A few odd responses, from a few very odd people,
slowly filtered through, but there was nobody who
really caught my attention.
I was losing interest in the whole idea, until up
popped a picture. Not a particularly brilliant photo
but the bio stood out as being OK. No bullshit or
fancy claims, just a normal Yorkshire girl. The best
thing about her was that she liked rock music, liked
motorcycles and seemed to like me.
I sent her my phone number and being somewhat
shy and nervous, was hoping that she wouldn't call.
But she did, and to my surprise I found that I could
talk to her without making a complete idiot out of
myself.
Something just felt right. We agreed to meet up at
the romantic setting of the Tesco Supermarket in

Wrexham on a Saturday night. The moment I saw her I was smitten.

The best thing about this girl, apart from being bloody gorgeous with a wonderful Yorkshire accent, was that she didn't mess with my mind. No mind games just straightforward talk, that I didn't have to decipher or get confused about. Exactly what I needed.

I had already decided that women like this simply didn't exist. I had convinced myself that they were all manipulative, scheming harpies with a hidden agenda.

It took me a long time to stop thinking this way. Nobody had ever shown me so much unconditional love and attention. Here I was with the girl of my dreams, everything I had ever wanted, a gorgeous, sexy, and fun to be with goddess. I couldn't believe it had finally happened. Because of this lack of belief, I panicked and ran away. Twice.

My daughter had been taken away by my ex wife to live in France, without either my knowledge or consent. I was in a new family, with two young kids, in a place that was alien to me. The stupid, nonsensical part of my brain went into overload.

I can't make sense of what I must have been thinking because it's a blur. I reckon it was all a bit too much for my mind to process and I just flipped.

The most amazing thing about it all was that my new woman came and found me, brought me home and forgave me. I'll never forget that. I love her more than ever.

She's still bloody gorgeous too.

I know that I must be difficult to live with. I am possessed by the constant worry of it all becoming too much for my long suffering wife. I never do anything with the intention of causing her pain or grief. I just get it wrong sometimes, despite my best intentions.

My own thoughts make me paranoid and I try to overcompensate if I think I've done something wrong, not done enough or made her unhappy. It's mentally exhausting at times, but I try to be the best husband that I can be.

Despite most people's ideas about bikers being drunken womanisers, I have only had 3 sexual partners my whole life and been married to each one. To me, sex is a very loving and spiritual thing. Without love it is an empty act. I don't understand how anyone can have sex with a prostitute, in the full knowledge that they don't even want be there. You might as well buy a blow up doll. Maybe it's just me that thinks this way.

I think my biggest problem comes from being mentally tortured and manipulated by people in my past. It has left me feeling very insecure and with major trust issues, but life and love go on regardless.

It wasn't too long before I was back on two wheels. The missus loves bikes as much as I do and spotted a Kawasaki for sale in the local paper for a decent price. It turned out to be a GPZ 1000R.
 They're a little over complicated and dated but bordering on insane. It was extremely fast and powerful but still quite comfortable. Once I had removed the bloody awful 'Bad Boy' stickers, It looked great.
We decided to go to a bike rally. It was being held on the Wirral by the Snatch MCC and I distinctly remember thinking, and probably saying, "This is where I belong." Back amongst my people... bikers.
What I didn't know at the time was that I was about to meet some people who would become like a family to me and change my life forever.

I had been a supporter of Chester City football club for many years and, by a tangled set of circumstances, ended up managing and coaching the ladies reserve football squad.

I got to know the chairman of Chester City Ladies FC because of his shared interest in bikes and it turned out that he was in a bike club. I must admit that I had never heard of them before, but my curiosity had been tickled.

As it happened, that very club were attending a charity event at the pub where the ladies team went for after match refreshments. There was something about them. They were not like anything I had witnessed before. They had a togetherness and look about them that appealed to my old school biker ways. George pointed out the club president and enforcer, then told me a little about the club in that guarded way, that I have since learned to be the norm.

It wasn't until around a year later, that I would see them again in the middle of a field , all sat around a Volkswagen trike, enjoying the sun and a few beers. Being rather lacking in self confidence but lubricated with a couple of beers, I plucked up the courage to go and introduce myself. I could not have been made more welcome. Each of them shook my hand and said hello with genuine warmth and a welcoming smile.

A few weeks later, at another rally, I was having a top bar sewn onto my newly acquired leather waistcoat, to begin a prospective membership of my newly found bike club, soulmates and extended family. I was definitely who I was supposed to be again.

On another trip to peruse the unaffordable, at Bill Smith's Motorcycles, a gleaming black and rather space age looking machine caught my eye. It was a Honda VFR 800. It had an unusual style that appeared angular yet smooth and aerodynamic. I never needed an excuse to change bikes and the Kawasaki Z650 I was riding at the time was a bit old and troublesome. Pen hit paper and a few days later I found myself riding back to North Wales on my new steed.

I had never ridden a bike like this before. The V4 engine whirred like a turbine and released its spent gasses through an ART silencer, that had a weird, hollow sound. Everything about the bike felt different but good at the same time.

It boasted a single sided swinging arm, which gave the appearance, from one side at least, that the back wheel was floating in space. The engine had gear driven cams that produced some serious engine braking and it was my first bike that utilized fuel injection to get things moving.

I had entered the age of computerised motorcycles and modern things. I wasn't sure if I was totally comfortable with it all. However, it did everything it should do with ease and a certain degree of individuality. At least it was my favourite colour for bikes. Black.

My wife had recently passed her bike test and was riding a Suzuki Bandit 600. We decided to attend the 'Stormin' the Castle' rally, many miles away in County Durham, a trip of around 180 miles, mostly on motorways.
We were meeting another club member and his wife up there. They had already arrived in their barely roadworthy, hand painted Volkswagen Camper van, that was held together with some very dubious welding, rust, and sheer luck. It had A top speed of around 60 mph and it's driver's eyesight left a lot to be desired. When I asked him about how he coped with not being able to see very well, he told me that he used the bumps from the cats eyes to guide him.... Oh dear.
I personally found the whole rally a bit of an anti climax. There were lots of things to do and see there and a good atmosphere . Perhaps I just wasn't in the mood. This was not helped by the damp, drizzly weather which decided, during Saturday night, that things needed livening up a bit and became a full blown storm.
Sunday morning revealed a scene of devastation. It looked like people had pitched their tents directly behind a jumbo jet, just before take off. Luckily,

ours had survived intact.

It was still extremely windy, mixed with showers, and we had to make the long trip home. We each had a child on the back of the bikes and the weather was showing no signs of easing off.

It was a nightmare journey, with a constant gusting, side wind battering us all the way. Not a good feeling on two wheels.

By the time we got home, thankfully in one piece, we were exhausted. I think it took me about a week to thoroughly pull myself out of a fixed riding position, after being tensed up for about 4 hours solid on the motorway. We've never been back.

The VFR never missed a beat and joins the short list of bikes I wish I still owned. I'm not really a fan of plastic covered, sporty bikes or Hondas for that matter, but the VFR range (of which I have owned 3) are a breed apart. They will run forever and handle just about anything you throw at them with little or no complaint. Maybe a little boring at times but they are genuinely excellent machines.

Motorcycles are so well equipped as standard today.

When I first got into bikes you had to spend a small fortune to get any sort of decent performance out of your chosen machine.

If you wanted a bit more power there were conical K&N or S&B air filters, with their air corrector kits, full 4 into 1 exhaust systems, electronic ignition kits and specialist coils.

If you wanted better handling there were box section swinging arms, from the likes of Davida Moto or Metchamex, shock absorbers from Marzocchi and fork braces by Micron. If you wanted to stop with any sort of purpose, you had to invest in a full set of Goodridge, braided steel brake lines. Weather protection came in the form of fairings by Rickman. They were a huge, heavy pieces of fibreglass, that bolted to the front of your chosen bike. They made for terrible low speed handling and increased fuel consumption due to the added weight.

If you were very rich, you could invest in a whole new frame from Harris, or a complete engine tuning kit from Yoshimura or Moriwaki.

If you were mega rich and of little taste, there was the exotic option of the Bimota range. These were standard Japanese bikes given a complete makeover by crazy Italians.

If you owned a 2 stroke bike, there were expansion pipes and engine porting to be done. It was often the case that some bikes got tuned to such a degree as to render them almost unrideable. It was sometimes more luck than knowledge which would lead to finding the right balance.

The list was inexhaustible and it was rare to see any bike in it's standard form.

I remember Chester's streets being populated by Kawasaki Z650s, which nearly always boasted a 2/4 seat, S&B filters and an Alpha 4 into 1 exhaust. Loud as hell and great fun, ridden by lads with fringed leather jackets, dirty jeans, Ashman boots and long greasy hair.... or was that me ?

One of the things about being a biker in the 80's was that we were classed as antisocial troublemakers and this suited me fine. It meant that people left me alone and gave me space. Being an introvert, this was exactly what I wanted.

I'm not really antisocial, I'm just very picky about who I choose to spend time with. I actually feel a lot better surrounded by those I know to be ruthless, violent, crazy bastards, who would quite happily shoot me if I crossed the line, simply because you know exactly where you stand with those guys. You don't really get that anywhere outside of the biker world.

There is a Buddhist saying which reads :

'I am not what you think I am... you are what you think I am.'

Read it a few times.
The best thing about that saying is that I honestly don't worry about what you think.
I'm one of the good guys by the way... honestly.

CHAPTER 8

'*Mental illness*

People assume you aren't sick
unless they see the sickness on your skin
like scars forming a map of all the ways you're
hurting.

My heart is a prison of Have you trieds?
Have you tried exercising? Have you tried eating
better?
Have you tried not being sad, not being sick?
Have you tried being more like me?
Have you tried shutting up?

Yes, I have tried. Yes, I am still trying,
and yes, I am still sick.

Sometimes monsters are invisible, and
sometimes demons attack you from the inside.
Just because you cannot see the claws and the
teeth
does not mean they aren't ripping through me.
Pain does not need to be seen to be felt.

Telling me there is no problem
won't solve the problem.

This is not how miracles are born.
This is not how sickness works.'

— Emm Roy, The First Step.

I think bikers should become the new government. We have little time for bullshit, liars, red tape or propaganda. We live by our word and respect those who show us the same in return. If something needs sorting out it gets done. If there's a problem, we'll have a quick meeting, take a vote and act accordingly. We are accepting and tolerant of whatever, race, religion, sexual orientation or opinions you may have , as long as it doesn't cause suffering to anyone else.

If somebody is in need, or in danger, we will drop everything to help.

But the most important thing you need to understand, is that we will do this without any thought for reward or recognition. Our reason are because it's the right thing to do. Not out of any need to boost the ego. No hidden agendas.

This is exactly what is missing in the greedy, self centred and uncaring society of today. It's all about

151

money and self promotion, regardless of who suffers as a consequence.

The justice system would be a whole lot simpler. If somebody takes away another's rights or freedom, then they automatically lose those rights themselves and will be punished according to their crime.
Bike thieves will be hung by the testicles until they promise never to do it again. But probably longer, with weights attached.

Whenever I travel abroad to, so called, third world countries, I always feel more at home than living in the United Kingdom. The reason for this is because, despite the people being materially poor, they are far richer in love. They look out for each other and have time for family and friends. Although they have very little to give, they would give it to you regardless, if you were in need.
It's not until the television starts making people believe they should have more of the things they don't really need, that it all starts to go wrong.
Bikers are at their best in each other's company with a few beers. You won't see us sat around watching TV or drinking at the latest trendy bar. We are people of simple tastes and pleasures. Quite low maintenance really.

I mentioned earlier about being very much in touch with my mortality. It's an unfortunate, but all too regular, part of this lifestyle, that we are going to lose people close to us on the road or see friends hurt or disabled. It happens to people in all walks of life but more so for us 2 wheeled road users, compared to the relative safety of 4.

I've lost count of friends and acquaintances killed or injured. Some due to other road users and some due entirely to their own overconfidence in their, or their bikes, abilities. Some are also down to plain stupidity.

Even when I hear about the death of a rider completely unknown to myself it makes me feel cold, but helps to remind me to take that extra bit of care.

If ever you witness a biker funeral and wonder why there are so many people there, or such a huge procession of bikes, it may surprise you to know that a lot of those people have never even met the deceased, but they know them in spirit and have a common bond.

The unfortunate reality of riding a motorcycle, in today's traffic, is that it is almost guaranteed, at various points during the trip, there will be a near miss.

I find more and more that, instead of just concentrating on where I'm going and what I'm doing, I am having to do it for everyone else. It all becomes a game of dodge the idiot.

There are a lot of good drivers out there, but today's cars are so full of entertainment systems, touch screen navigation and no end of flashing lights with associated beeps that it is far to easy for drivers to get distracted. Add to the mix being told that your car will do everything for you, including braking if something gets in it's way and you have a recipe for inattentivness and lack of concentration. You might not believe this but try riding a bike or travelling pillion and you'll soon see what I mean.

I notice these things when behind the wheel too. The highway is a very dangerous place if you don't have your wits about you.

During the 80's and 90's, if you asked any biker which car they took most care around, you always got the same answer... Volvos. The reason for this was simple.

Back then Volvo advertised their cars as the safest vehicle in the World and they probably were. They were built like tanks and had every modern safety feature available, but this made the drivers of these heavyweight Swedish lumps feel indestructible and they drove accordingly.

You will still find us taking a little more care around certain brands of motor vehicle, usually BMW or Audi, but my personal favourite is the 10 year old Nissan Micra. Usually driven by persons in their twilight years and only used for a trip to the supermarket or church on Sundays. They are given a very wide berth indeed, along with burgundy Ford Fiestas.

Joking aside, with inattentive drivers, potholes the size of small ponds and diesel from overfilled tanks spilled onto the roads, life on two wheels has become more survival than fun.
If we hit something we fall off, if you hit us from the side we lose a leg, if you hit us from behind we'll probably break our necks, if you spill diesel on the road we'll slide and crash and if you throw your cigarette stump out of your car window you will blind or burn us. Oh yes, those things that fly up of the road and crack windscreens ?... that's called my face. But we still do it. Maybe it's the thought of a sudden traumatic death that makes us feel alive. I'm always buzzing when I kick down that side stand after a bit of wind therapy and arrive at my destination intact.

I watched something recently on Television about how the human brain works and it was rather worrying to say the least. I have found this to be the case on a number of occasions in everyday life and it happens more often than you might think.

Imagine if you suddenly decide to go looking for something that you haven't seen in a while, a screwdriver perhaps. You have a mental image of that particular tool. It's about a foot long with a yellow handle. You know you have one, it's in the shed somewhere and you go to look for it. The problem is that it actually has a red handle but you'd forgotten that.

You find the tool bag and rummage through it... The screwdriver is there, right in front of you but your brain refuses to see it because it expects it to have a yellow handle. That is what it's specifically searching for and everything else gets dismissed. How many times have you found something that you were looking for previously in exactly the same place you had searched for it, but when you are no longer looking for it ? Your brain no longer has that specific image to blind you and 'It was there all the time'.

The same thing happens with a lot of drivers, those who don't have motorcycles in their lives especially. When waiting at a busy junction, for instance, looking for other vehicles coming from each side, their brain expects to see cars, vans or trucks. If

they do not expect to see a bike, their brain simply won't see it until it crashes into the side of the car. The expression uttered by many drivers following a collision with a motorcycle... "Sorry mate I didn't see you." Is often the truth.
Always remember this while riding and expect the worst.

It's not always other road users of course.
 Testosterone and bad judgement have a lot to answer for.
I worked with a lad at the Royal Mail, called Alistair, who owned a couple of bikes. One of these bikes was a pristine, 6 cylinder, Honda CBX 1000. A very powerful machine at the time. For reasons, known only to himself, he decided to let his brother use it on a trip between Wrexham and Whitchurch. Just a few minutes into the journey there are a few sets of very tight bends situated on hills, which are well known accident blackspots. Apparently his brother went speeding ahead, out of site, perhaps showing off a little, only for Alistair to reach one of these bends to find little pieces of his motorcycle and brother spread across the road following a collision with an articulated wagon. The impact had been so great that his body had literally disintegrated. I believe Alistair never rode a bike again after that.

One quite recent accident, if the term accident is appropriate for something totally avoidable, involved a group of what are known to us old school bikers as 'power rangers', on high performance machinery with matching leathers and helmets. They were riding along a countryside road as if it were a Grand Prix track, showing off to each other and taking stupid risks. Another group of riders were heading towards them, riding sensibly and keeping to their side of the road. The power rangers rounded a bend too fast and were unable to keep to their side of the road, due to excessive speed and lack of common sense. The resulting collision resulted in the decapitation of one of the innocent riders and the maiming or death of a couple more. The scene was described by the emergency services as utter carnage.

I know of a few instances where a rider has gone into a sharp bend too close to the centre line and had his head removed by an oncoming truck.

There is a tale of two bikers on the motorway that didn't realise how quickly a wagon had stopped in front of them, resulting in the top half of their bodies being found inside the truck while the rest was underneath.

There are enough horror stories to fill a book on their own, but it's all a bit too morbid.

What really amazes me are motorcyclists that think they are indestructible. You know the ones. You see them as soon as it's warm enough, riding high powered bikes in a vest top, shorts, and trainers. The average human can jog at around 8 mph... If you trip and fall at this speed it will hurt, you'll have cuts and grazes plus a few good bruises. So what do you think will happen at 30, 50, 80 mph? You'll lose skin down to the bone, break a few bones, damage various internal organs, lose a fair bit of blood, spend the next few weeks picking gravel out of your skin and quite possibly die. But that's ok because your wearing 500 quids worth of race replica helmet. Must be safe.

It really doesn't matter how much gear you wear sometimes. The impact of a motorcycle accident often tears the aorta (the main blood vessel from the heart). A motorcyclist can get up from a crash, apparently uninjured, only to drop dead a few seconds later.

It would be easy to allow all this negativity to stop me doing what I love and hang up my leather jacket for good. It doesn't help when my friendly little mental demons are experts at planting ifs, whats and maybes into my consciousness. They will find a million reasons not to do something with a trillion possible outcomes if I do. If they had their way I would be living a life wrapped in bubble wrap, never leaving the safety of my bed and drinking chamomile tea.

The secret is to let them have their playing out time and, just like little children, they will get tired and give up. I know they'll be back later with renewed vigour and a plethora of freshly imagined scenarios, but that's their thing and I have mine. I've learnt nowadays, with a modicum of success, to just switch channels and let the 'Hyperactive Demon Channel' play away to itself in the background. It's a pity I can't always find the remote.

When people say, "Don't dwell on things." or, "Try not to overthink things.", it's not a choice that I have. It's part of me that I have accepted as being a normal feature of my existence.

What I have discovered is that, by accepting this, I can use the mental mayhem as an aid to creativity. It's rather like having the whole catalogue of Google images, iTunes and the Oxford English Dictionary on tap. You just have to learn to live life as if you spend all day living on the central reservation of the M6 motorway, during rush hour, on a bank holiday weekend. There is more than enough information available, it's just a matter of picking good stuff out of the mayhem.

Now I let it stream through a pen or keyboard. Both are my pressure valve.

Another byproduct of experiencing everything, all of the time is that, whether you want to be or not, you become an empath. An empath feels the emotions of others as strongly as if they were their own. If people close to me are happy, then I am happy. Of course it works both ways.
I only have to be within a few feet of somebody to feel the buzz of energy from them, be that anger, worry, sadness or bliss. There are people I can sit in total silence with (a rare few) and know that they also feel content to do the same. On the other hand there are people that I just want to get as far away from as possible, as soon as possible.
This comes in very useful in my line of work as a Security Officer.
Being able to read energy is an invaluable tool when dealing with the public. If something doesn't feel right, that's the energy telling you something. It is nearly always right.
While out riding, there have been numerous times when I changed which route I take for no other reason, other than something told me not to go that way. Of course I'll never know if I avoided something bad because I wasn't there, and I've never ignored it to find out. Some might say that

bikers have a sixth sense, I think we just read the energy better. Maybe without even realising what we're doing.

As for my merry go round of motorcycles, I had decided to swap the Honda VFR 800 for a big ugly BMW tourer. A BMW K1100LT to be precise.
This thing was basically a bike, with a car engine attached, and a huge fairing which had a screen that could be raised or lowered electronically. Despite being extremely comfortable it had the strange knack of taking away all sensation of speed. The fairing worked so well, aerodynamically that, regardless of how fast you were travelling, you were sat in a pocket of still air. Along with this came a very unusual effect produced by the screen. When it was fully extended, it created some sort of turbulence that actually pushed the rider from the rear, which is a little unnerving whilst travelling forwards.
The biggest problem with lacking all feeling of forwards momentum was that I would find myself approaching bends much faster than I thought and having to lean, the huge lump of a bike, over at crazy angles in order to negotiate the turn. There were many moments of buttock clenching and curse words whispered to myself inside my helmet.

However, this was way up on my list of most boring motorcycles ever. It was one of those bikes which did everything that is was built to do, in that effortless way with which the Germans have become masters, but in a soulless, empty fashion. It had to go.

I swapped it for another BMW. One that sent my right hand to sleep on motorways. It was a quirky but capable lump with a 'boxer' style twin cylinder engine. If you sat on the bike and blipped the throttle, it would twitch to the right. It looked weird too.

The BMW R1100/850R series are superb bikes that handle the twisty bits better than any bike I have ever owned. They have big bags of torque and will take you wherever you want to go without a worry. They're just so bloody complicated.

My 850cc version needed a new throttle cable; never a big issue on most bikes, so I had a look on YouTube for a few hints on how to go about it. It took 2 fully qualified BMW mechanics, in a fully fitted workshop, about 4 hours to complete the task. I have limited tools, an open driveway and very little time for the boffins, at the Bayerische Motoren Werke design departments, sick sense of humour. Ridiculous is too nice a word.

Now that I'm past the age of 50, I always look at how comfortable a bike will be.

Hip cramp is one of the worst things associated with age related lack of supple joints. If ever you see a biker pulling away from a set of traffic lights with his leg stretched out in front of him, it's because he's in bloody agony.

You put your legs down as you reach a standstill and patiently await the green light, click the gearbox into first, slowly pull away and lift your legs back onto the footpegs. Then it hits. It's like you've been stabbed in the hip with large fork and King Kong is slowly twisting it. The only way to get through the pain is either swearing profusely through gritted teeth or sticking out the affected limb in a rather comical fashion.

The other option is to buy a cruiser with forward footpegs. The only issue with this type of set up is that if you remove your feet from the pegs at any great speed, it becomes somewhat difficult to get them back on. The problem increases as you get faster and is absolutely hilarious to your fellow riding buddies.

It amuses me when a group of us have been on a long ride and get off our bikes, only to perform stretching, groaning, rubbing bits and making various wincing noises. Oh for the days of youthfulness when the only thing that hurt were skinned knuckles from slipping spanners or getting reminders for your road tax, MOT and insurance just before pay day.

Insurance used to be very simple. It was just a matter of paying a single premium that enabled you to ride any bike up to a certain cc limit, regardless of how you much you had modified it. This was great unless you were the owner of a Honda CB900. This was because one of the categories was, 'any bike up to 900cc'. Anything after that was in the unlimited cc bracket and was much more expensive. The Honda had a displacement of 901cc. Never mind.
Nowadays insurance is a minefield created by companies to confuse you with overcomplicated policy rules, designed to give them an excuse not to pay out if you make a claim. "Oh... I see here that you didn't inform us about changing your mirrors... sorry sir we can't possibly honour our part of the contract. Even though you haven't made a claim for 30 years and paid us thousands. Sorry. Please call again."

The modern motorcycle throws up a number of problems when it comes to regular, DIY maintenance.

Most bikes today have a brain. A little metal box full of stuff that I regard as magic and witchcraft. This Pandora's box of electrical thingies, apparently, controls everything from how much fuel reaches the engine to how fast your indicators flash.

I used to understand how things worked and therefore knew how to fix them. Armed with just a Halfords socket set, a few spanners, a couple of screwdrivers and a large hammer, I could bodge and curse my way through almost anything that needed doing on my old bikes. The only things that ever stopped me were Philips head screws made out of the softest metal known to man, seized exhaust bolts and getting distracted by something else. This would result in the tools I required to finish the job being whisked away by the shed gremlins and hidden until I was no longer looking for them and had bought another one. The gremlins never leave and are companions for life,which is why I now own approximately fifteen 10mm spanners.

Replacing the chain and sprockets was always a good bet for receiving some kind of, tool induced, injury. A lot of moving parts, covered in oil, requiring varying degrees of force to facilitate their removal is always a good recipe for an open wound covered in filthy black grease.

The bolt holding the front sprocket in place
presented the ideal opportunity for the creation of
 previously unheard swear words. Along with the
curses were a generous helping of cuts and
bruises, on several parts of the anatomy, from
when whatever you were employing to loosen said
nut, slipped off under force and hit whatever was in
it's path. Usually a shin bone.
Then there are the horror stories of fingers trapped
between the chain and rear sprocket but I find it
hard to even think about that.

Yet out of all the DIY mechanical odds and ends
that cause distress, nothing holds the title of
'Absolute Bastard' more than the Suzuki GS model
airbox.
This is the place just behind the carburettors, on
Suzuki's four cylinder models, where the air filter
lives and breathes. If any job needs doing on the
carbs it has to be removed. Not a problem you
might think, except for the fact that the guys in the
factory, somewhere in Japan, were quietly
sniggering to themselves while designing this
particular part.
The first thing you must do is loosen the rubber
manifolds that fit onto the rear of the carburettors
and move the whole airbox backwards. Bearing in
mind the degree of rearward movement permitted

by the motorcycle frame is approximately half an inch and the manifolds are made of rubber, therefore somewhat elastic. Plus there are four of them, all attempting to remain attached to the rear of the carbs despite your best efforts. Add to this the necessity of wiggling the airbox around in order to remove it from the side of the bike, which requires the same sort of dexterity and cunning as solving a Rubic Cube, blindfolded, with no hands, while drunk. This wiggling backward and forward allows the cheeky little manifolds to keep popping back onto the carbs whenever they feel like and usually have the effect of sending the owner away for a cup of tea, or large shot of whiskey, before he finally cracks and finds the sledgehammer or a box of matches.

But if you thought that was bad, try putting one back on. One of the many unusual uses of Vaseline, and it requires the arms of an octopus.

Nobody ever told us how to do stuff. All we had was not enough money to pay a proper mechanic and a Haynes manual. Plus, more often than not, a few left over nuts and bolts on the garage floor, that obviously weren't important.

Nothing much compares to the feeling of accomplishment that follows fixing something that would have cost a small fortune to have done professionally. Especially when the bike fires into life and nothing explodes or makes the wrong noises. You might be covered in oil and grease, missing various tools and have a couple of fingers missing, but it was all worth it.

One way that my ADD affects me is that I find it very difficult to perform any task if others are watching or if I even think they are. I can be perfectly competent at whatever that task might be, but will become a useless bag of nerves in the presence of a voyeur. Put me in a garage on my own and I will strip down and rebuild an engine without a problem. Put someone in there with me and I start making mistakes.

If I know somebody is going to be there I begin to overthink the whole process and imagine every possible way to get things wrong. This applies to driving more than anything. Instead of just concentrating on what I'm doing, I worry about what my passenger is thinking and believe they are critical of the way I do things. This makes me very tense, nervous, and causes me to make mistakes. I'm a much better driver when flying solo.

When I first started riding with the Evicted MCC, I would often make an excuse not to ride together on the way to a rally because I thought they would be judging the way I rode and I became afraid of making a mistake or not being able to keep up. It's a side effect of the overactive brain creating scenarios of possible failure.

I believe, my childhood experiences involving the absence of any communication from my parents, unless it was of the negative kind, hasn't helped much.

99% of verbal communication during my childhood was being told off for something or criticism, so that what I learned to expect from everyone.

I also have very guilty conscience. My brain has thought about a million ways to get into trouble so feels bad for the thoughts alone. It doesn't help that I blush redder than a baboon's backside over the slightest thing.

Since gaining an understanding of why these things happen, I manage to kick myself up the arse and get on with it to some extent. However, that little devil will sometimes pop up onto my shoulder and whisper into my ear, "You're not doing very well are you?".

I keep trying to brush him away but he's a persistent little bugger, with lots of mates.

CHAPTER 9

'Some of us can begin to heal the damage people have done to us by escaping the situation, but some of us need more than that. Tattoos make statements that need to be made. Or hide things that are no one's business. Your scars are battle wounds, but you don't see them that way. Yet.'
— **Tammara Webber, Breakable**

What makes us endure the discomfort of getting a tattoo? The initial pain, waiting for it to scab over, it starting to heal and itching like hell. Never mind spending a small fortune for the privilege. It does make me wonder why I bother, but I still want more. Lots more. It's highly addictive you know.

When I summoned up the courage to get my first bit of ink, a small Celtic design on my upper arm, tattoos were still seen as a little taboo. This was one of my main reasons for getting one.

Some psychologists suggest that tattoos are a way of rebelling against your parents, so perhaps that also had something to do with it. Whatever the reason I had this burning desire to get some body art.

I have to admit to feeling rather disappointed at the way in which tattoos have become fashionable and such a commonly accepted thing nowadays. I blame celebrities and the sheep that follow them. If David Beckham gets a tattoo, every young lad decided that if they got a similar one, they would look just like him, get a wife like Victoria and become instantly rich. Didn't work though, did it ?

It's a rare bond between you and your tattooist. They are about to shave part of your anatomy, cause you pain, scar you for life, hopefully spell things correctly then ask for loads of money. Talk about trust.

The guy who first pushed a needle into my skin was a real character. He had served his time tattooing Hells Angels in Holland and relaxed by chain smoking while fishing for sharks.

He had a look about him that was somewhere between Keith Richards and The Fonz, after a weekend of heavy drinking. He appeared to be about 70 years old but was probably only about 45. I had several tattoos done by him and on one memorable occasion a middle aged woman popped her head around the door to express her concerns regarding the chances of her daughter contracting

something like AIDS if she got a tattoo. His reply
has stuck with me since...

"look missus, if I was to fuck your daughter she
wouldn't get AIDS, now get out of my shop." The
look on her face was a picture.

I had my nose pierced in the same shop and,
although I liked the look of it, it just became too
much bother. It never felt comfortable or fully
healed. The same thing happened when I had my
lip pierced recently. I reckon my body simply rejects
foreign object that it doesn't think should be there.

I don't think there is anything more beautiful than
thoughtfully inked tattoos on a woman. Maybe it's
just a fetish of mine... who knows.

Personally, if I was a rich man, there wouldn't be
much space left on this old body. Every tattoo on
my body signifies a time in my life, like a history
picture book. They all have meaning and I regret
none of them. The most pleasurable thing about my
tattoos is that my mother hates them, which is
always a massive bonus.

On the subject of money (vaguely). I work in a
industry that doesn't pay a great deal. I have a
whole load of bills to pay each month but we get by
OK. We have a roof over our heads, we each have
a nice bike, we eat well and have a bit left over to
enjoy ourselves.

I have nothing against anyone who has a lot more money than me and it's absolutely nothing to do with me how they spend it. But one thing is an undeniable truth. All the money in the world will not make you a biker.

Yes, you can go out and buy the latest badass looking Harley Davidson and every shiny accessory to stick on it. You can get the 500 quid leather jacket, 300 quid boots and a few hundred quid more on whatever you reckon makes you look the part. Unfortunately this won't get the result you're looking for. It will just make you look exactly what you are. A fake.

I'm sure you've seen these guys, usually of retirement age, chugging around on very loud bikes, with gleaming chrome and fancy paint. They won't smile because they think it's not the cool thing to do and it makes them look mean. They won't acknowledge other riders, because they just don't get it and think they're better than them. You'll find them at biker cafe's, sat on their own, next their machine, thinking others are admiring it. The truth is, we're not even slightly impressed and muttering, "Oh for fucks sake." to ourselves.

I can't help feeling sorry for this race of motorcyclists because they will never understand what we've got and, most of all, they think it's not cool to ask.

One of the most genuine characters I have ever
known was Biff.
A man with a serious bike obsession and addiction,
but with the innocence of a child. He cared not for
the biker image and followed the philosophy of,
'Who cares what it looks like, as long as it does the
job'.
Biff had a permanent air of bewilderment about
him, as if he wasn't quite sure what was going on,
but he just didn't care. Motorcycles were his life and
everything revolved around them. He talked about
nothing else, had an encyclopaedic knowledge of
everything related to two wheel travel and could tell
you what bike was coming just by the sound it
made. The best thing about conversations with Biff
were the added bike sounds, which were always
spot on.
This is a guy who rode around a roundabout about
20 times because he liked the sound of his 600cc,
single cylinder Kawasaki. He set fire to his shoes
after removing the silencers from his BMW to see
what it sounded like, wrapped them in gaffer tape
and kept riding. A proper nutcase.
Biff didn't drink when I first met him, but during one
rally weekend, he succumb to the demon alcohol.
He retired to his tent and spent the rest of the
afternoon laughing and shouting "Esmeralda...

Esmeralda.... come and give me a blowjob."
Nobody knew who Esmeralda was but we all
steered well clear of his tent, just in case of
mistaken identity.

His childlike personality and naivety cost him dear
when an ogre of a woman got her claws into him
and got pregnant, only to take him for everything
she could.

I've no idea where Biff is nowadays, but have no
doubt he will reappear one day to carry on talking
about his most recent bike and close call with
death, as if it were only yesterday.

Another great personality from my past was Spong.
It was actually his surname but doubled as a
nickname. Not really sure how we came to be
friends , it just sort of happened.

Spong was one of those natural freaks of nature
which occurs when the world decides it needs a bit
of help.

Standing at around 6 foot 5 inches and built like a
prize bull, he rode a tiny Honda CB550 four, that he
made look like a 50cc moped.

He used to work in the coal mines and saved the
lives of countless miners by becoming a human pit
prop when one of the tunnels started to cave in. He
spoke of this as if it were just a daily event, with the
humility and modesty to match.

He had moved to the outskirts of Chester from
Stoke on Trent, following an incident when some
Asian youths had tried to steal his bike, that is until
he opened his flat window and shot one of them in
the leg with a crossbow.

He lived on a canal, in a narrow boat, with his
girlfriend and rode his bike up a plank to store it on
board. Not an easy task to master and one that you
certainly don't want to get wrong.

Despite his size and having hands the size of snow
shovels, he made a living by creating incredibly
delicate jewellery, in the form of famous aircraft, to
sell to a local aerospace company. Tiny, cufflink
size executive jets, spitfires and mosquito bombers
in gold and silver. It still amazes me how he did it.
He had this knack of finding strange and remote
places of interest, that nobody else seemed to
know existed. He would say, "Fancy going for a ride
out?" and a few hours later, via various country
lanes and tracks, we'd happen upon a long
forgotten piece of history.

One such road trip ended in the discovery of a
huge, derelict stately home and gardens. Our
arrival was heralded by hundreds of crows taking to
the skies from their, rarely disturbed, perches
amongst the decaying ruins. How the hell he knew
it was there, let alone how to get there, I'll never

177

know. It was somewhere in the Midlands
apparently.
The last I heard from Spong was many years ago
when he found work near London, untied the
narrow boat and chugged away along the maze of
waterways with a Kawasaki, Z900 precariously
perched on the bow.

I've always managed to get along with people,
despite my fondness for avoiding them. I try not to
give anyone a reason to dislike me but sometimes
things just go horribly wrong.
Maybe not with people, but it would appear that the
odd motorcycle doesn't like me at all.

I owned an old Suzuki GS850 that I bought off my
mate Grizzler. I have always liked four cylinder
Suzies, so I decided to make it a custom bike
project.
It had served him well for many years but, as soon
as it was wrenched away from it's loving owner, it
decided that it wasn't going to be my friend. In fact
it hated me.
I stripped it down, painted the frame, polished and
painted the engine, repainted the wheels, treated it
to new mudguards, a handmade seat from
Portugal, new lights, handlebars and a custom
petrol tank. I painstakingly wrapped the exhaust

pipes in titanium, heat dispersing wrap, added some custom silencers and treated it to a satin black paint job with fine white pinstripe designs. It was looking mighty fine indeed.... It simply refused to start.

I left the bike overnight, hoping that it would calm down and think about what it had done. On my return I discovered that the new petrol tank had leaked, ruining the new paint and dripping petrol everywhere. I later found out that the tank was completely knackered, having been repaired with body filler, in about 20 places. Body filler doesn't like petrol very much, so I had to get another tank. The worst thing was that I had sold the original tank, thinking I wouldn't be needing it again. Another lesson learned.

The electrical system refused to let anything work without stopping something else from functioning and, even when I managed to get it started, it just wouldn't run properly.

The most annoying thing about it all was that I hadn't really changed much from when I acquired the thing, but it just wouldn't play nicely.

I would pull onto the road and open the throttle, only to be treated to a symphony of pops, crackles, splutters and little more. The one time that I managed to ride the unruly contraption any sort of distance it tried to kill me.

I had used exactly the same size fasteners to attach the front mudguard as the originals and I had a new front tyre fitted, of the same make and type as the old one. Somehow, due to the tyre expanding when it got warm (as all tyres do) it made contact with a bolt on the underside of the mudguard and cut a deep groove into the tyre. I was lucky it didn't just disintegrate, with the inevitable and rather painful results.

I dismantled, cleaned and re-jetted the carburettors more times than I care to wipe from my memory, but that old GS dug her heels in and folded her arms across her chest. I'm sure if it had been able to, it would have thrown a tantrum on the floor and arched it's back if any attempt was made to pacify the petulant shrew.

It had become my nemesis. After hundreds of hours of work, lack of sleep and quite a few quid, I gave up. She was swapped for an old Honda CBX 750. I didn't really want a Honda, but I did want some sleep.

I have visions of it's new owner, hunched in the corner of his garage, quietly sobbing to himself and peaking through his fingers to see if it's still there, contemplating it's next move. I keep finding bits of it in my shed and a cold shudder runs through my body in remembrance of what I would rather forget.

I had a short affair with another chopper. I bought it from a guy in the club, now an ex member. It was an old Honda 750 four of 1970s vintage. A traditional chopper with hardtail frame, extended forks and huge 'apehanger' (self explanatory) handlebars.

It was fine to ride until anything past 60 mph, when it became comparable to running into a gale force wind holding a 6 foot square piece of hardboard to your chest.

Going around bends gave the impression that the back wheel was attached by a number of loose elastic bands and would catch up with the rest of the bike when it felt like it.

A marvellous innovation by Honda, at the time, was the automatic drive chain lubrication system. This was basically a hole in the engine that dripped a small amount of oil onto the drive chain, but also onto the wife's newly block paved drive. It had to go.

Another swap later and I became the owner of a truly wonderful wee beastie. The Yamaha TRX 850. I have rarely enjoyed riding something quite as much as this marvellous contraption.

Yamaha had taken the twin cylinder engine from their very popular, but rather dull TDM 850 (sounds like tedium quite suitably), played around with it's innards and stuck it in a triangular design frame that made it handle like it was on rails. With a decent pair of exhaust silencers it sounded like a big Ducati and was often confused for one, just by the beautiful sound it produced.

I loved the thing to bits. I scraped the sole off my boots on roundabouts and the throttle responded with a crispness and thumping torque that could raise a smile from the most depressing of days. But as fate would have it, my missus was unable to ride her bike due to an operation and needed to ride pillion. This was not a bike created with a passenger in mind, so being the caring, loving, unselfish, perfect and modest husband, it went to join the growing list of bikes past in order to get something more suitable for wifey transportation. However I still want one. They are unlike anything else churned out by the Japanese industrial Machine. One day maybe. I'll write a nice letter to Santa.

I swapped it for a Yamaha FZR 1000 EXUP. A soulless sports bike that I never really got on with at all.

Rallies and bike shows still went on. I'm a lot better at controlling my inner party animal nowadays, but my problem lies with the safety cut off button. I never used to have one at all and spent many a late night technicolour yawning outside my tent, while the missus partially undressed me and dragged me inside.

One particular bike show, on the Isle of Anglesey in Wales, involved a group of, scantily clad, young ladies promoting Jaegermeister, which is basically alcoholic cough medicine. They were selling it for a pound and serving it in test tubes. It seemed like a good idea at the time, as such things do, until myself and my buddy Trash, found ourselves performing synchronised puking within crawling distance of our tents. I think the women just left us to get on with it that time.

Now I have a relatively well functioning safety cut of button. However, the demons are still able to distract me now and then, so I forget it's there at all. One such night was a club trip to a bar in Whitchurch.

The night started well but the sheer variety of weird and wonderful beverages to sample was simply too much to resist. We drank most of them. Well somebody had to!

There were Jaeger Bombs, Fire Bombs, Skittle Bombs, Amaretto Bombs, Tequila Shots complete with worms and various nuclear strength draught ciders and beers. How I managed to stay upright and compos mentis still remains a mystery.

The highlight of the night was one of the lads finishing a pint of beer only to refill the glass immediately with his own vomit. Apparently it's a talent. To be honest I have never seen my buddy in anything like that state before. He is one of those really annoying people that can imbibe enough during the evening to see most of us rushed off to hospital with alcohol poisoning and still wake up the next day, before any of us, fresh as a daisy and full of energy.

Biker event drunks tend to fall into a number of categories…

There's the happy drunk, who dances like nobody's watching, tries to get everyone else dancing and loves everyone. Often seen attempting to climb the centre pole of the marquee in a semi naked state. He'll sing on his way back to his tent where he collapses into a deep snoring sleep.

The sleepy drunk will be passed out, slumped over a table with his buddies balancing empty cans and bottles on his head. He will wake up at around 0430 and wonder where everyone has gone. Alternatively the sleepy drunk will say to his mates, "Just going for a pee lads" and you'll trip over him some time later after he's nodded off in the middle of the field, usually when it's started to rain.

The angry drunk will start to stagger around the dance floor and believe that everyone else if bumping into *him*. He doesn't get very far because, unbeknownst to him, he's been spotted some time ago and as soon as he starts to kick off, he'll be whisked away and quietly advised to go to bed or be put there under duress.

Bike revving drunks are a strange breed. For whatever reason possesses them, they are suddenly driven to find their keys, start up their bike and rev the bollocks off it, usually at 0230 in the morning, when everyone has just got to sleep. It is not uncommon for the culprit to have his keys confiscated and, if not responsive to polite requests for the ceasing of valve bouncing activities, a punch in the face.

Bonfire drunks are special type of rally goer. As soon as a bonfire is lit they are attracted to it by some primeval force and will move in and out of it's proximity, dependant on the fire's heat output. They will still be there when you wake up the next morning, sitting next to a few gently smoking embers and a mountain of beer cans, putting the world to rights. If they haven't been killed by shrapnel from carelessly discarded camping gas containers of course.

The over friendly drunk can be a problem. There are always one or two of these at every event.
His name is usually Nigel but will tell you he has a cool nickname, like 'Wolf', in an attempt to make himself appear interesting.
Always over 40, with breath that stinks of garlic and those little bits of frothy spit at the corners of his mouth when speaking to you.
Armed with tall tales of past motorcycling exploits and how his dad's second cousin won the senior TT in 1963. He'll usually just park himself at the end of a table where friends are enjoying their own company and immediately kill the mood, moving on to similar, unsuspecting tables when it becomes obvious that nobody wants to talk to him anymore.
His clothes have that smell of unaired dampness along with leather trousers that would probably look OK on anyone else but are offset by dirty white trainers. He'll be wearing a denim waistcoat, covered in hundreds of rally badges, with an iron on skull patch on the back and various hilarious (not) biker patches.
Homing in on anyone that appears to be alone or inadvertently makes eye contact, you will eventually

see him at the end of the night, sat next to a
sleeping drunk as if it's his best mate, still clutching
the same, half empty can of Carling lager.

His bike is a very low mileage Yamaha XV650
Dragstar with every bolt on chrome accessory
available, leather tassels on the luggage and a big
ugly screen. He puts it in all the custom bike shows
and never understands why it never wins a prize.
He'll go home and tell his mum all about what a
great weekend it was while she washes his back in
the bath.

Last but not least is the staring drunk. There you
are, minding your own business, watching the party
goers enjoying themselves. Then suddenly, out of
the corner of your eye, you see him staring straight
at you. It's as if you had murdered his entire family
last week and he wants revenge.

When he sees you've clocked him, he will hold the
stare for a second then look away slowly, but that's
not the end of it. It will happen several times during
the night. You begin to wonder what the hell his
problem is; 'do I know him from somewhere', 'Has
he mistaken me for someone else or did I actually
kill off his family last weekend ?'.

It reaches a point where you have to find out what
the problem is, so you wander across to confront
him, only to discover that he's one of the nicest

guys you've ever met and has no recollection of staring whatsoever, but people always think he is. Must be his natural demeanour.

Nowadays I fall into the category of, 'If I don't go to bed right now I'll be sorry'. Getting old you understand.

CHAPTER 10

'Trajectories aren't linear. Life's just a roller coaster. If you're getting a chance to do cool stuff, and it's varied stuff, just enjoy it. I guess I'm a believer in the randomness of life rather than it being a linear trajectory or an arc, a consistent smooth arc, towards anything.'
Riz Ahmed

After the discovery of my ADD/ADHD, I began to reflect back on my life and the events that steered my runaway train towards the present .
I tried to find a pattern or plan but there just wasn't one. Everything in my past has been a random set of events and continues to be so. The best thing about it is that I love it like that. Unplanned, unusual happenings, out of the blue. Let's face it, if you knew exactly what was going to happen every day, you'd soon get bored.
For some people, routine and similarity is their idea of heaven, but not for me thankyou very much.
My working days are very routine and boring, but I get paid for the drudgery. That's life unfortunately. If you want to live comfortably, you have to bite the bullet and get on with it.

The first time I have any recollection of something
weird happening was when I was just a little kid,
before I joined that brainwashing institution called
school.

Due to my Grandfather's poor health, my parents
had to sell their newly acquired house and move
into my Grandparent's pub, situated on Chester's
Town Hall Square, known as the Coach and
Horses. It's still there but altogether a much more
classy establishment.

I distinctly remember witnessing an event that I
could not have possibly seen at the time.

Looking out of the living room window, on the first
floor, I recollect in perfect detail, one of the street
lamps on the corner of St Werburgh street being on
fire and the Fire Brigade arriving on the scene to
extinguish it.

'Nothing unusual there', you might be thinking,
except that the firemen were wearing brass helmets
and the street lamp was burning gas.

This was approximately 1964 and due to fireman
receiving unwanted electroconvulsive therapy, via
the excellent conductive properties of a brass brain
covering when climbing a ladder directly towards
electrical cables, they stopped wearing them in the

1930's. Apart from this fact, I think it's fair to say that, by the 1960's, Chester had caught up with the rest of the modern World and were employing electricity, of the head frying kind, to light it's streets.

So where does this memory come from? I do have a particularly vivid imagination but at the ripe old age of 2 years old, I doubt that it was anywhere near developed enough to create such a scene.

Many years later, in our new home, I used to spend lots of time in the back garden.

When I wasn't burning stuff or causing my father to shout at me for waking him up after his night shift, I would imagine that I was a renowned archaeologist and dig random holes in the hope of finding a complete stegosaurus skeleton, or the tomb of a Roman Legionnaire.

Strangely enough I didn't find anything like that but what I did find, about 2 feet under the surface, was a stack of beautifully decorated, china dinner plates, in perfect condition. Makes about as much sense to me now as it did then. I find it hard to find any sort of explanation as to why anyone would feel the need to bury part of their best dinner service in the back garden of a modest semi detached property, on the outskirts of Chester. Unless they were put there with the sole intention of confusing any future, aspiring young archaeologists. In which case it worked perfectly. Nice one.

On reflection, it was more than likely my spinning top of a brain that created most of the random events.

An idea would pop into my head and that was it. I would launch myself into that thought without the aid of a safety net. I think this might be a family affliction.

My eldest brother was a master of the random act and the, 'What could possibly go wrong?' scenario. He accumulated a variety of minor injuries whilst pursuing this lifestyle, with the sort of innocence and positivity you only ever saw in small children or puppies. If it moved, he would fall off it or get knocked off. Simple as that. Horses, bicycles, you name it.

One such incident involved him colliding head on with a taxi whilst riding a pushbike, resulting in the performance of an airborne double somersault over the top of the taxi. Luckily this occurred outside the local hospital when he was on his way to start work there.

As a child I used to stay awake as long as I could , looking down the road for the bouncing walk of my big brother, often wearing an old Police cape, and huge boots, as he returned from one of his long trips at sea with the merchant navy.

He worked as a steward on the Queen Mary and would often bring home weird souvenirs from various parts of the world, including a huge teddy bear from Russia that made a spooky, screaming noise if you flipped him over. His name was Ivan and he was a bit scary.

I knew that when he was around there would be adventures to be had and trouble to get into.

A typical scenario would be trip somewhere miles away from home, where he would spend all his money on treats, leaving nothing left to pay for the bus fare home. This often meant a ten mile walk and whatever extra mischief could be accomplished along the way.

Nothing ever came as a surprise with big bruv. I expect our parents were in a constant state of disbelief and despair, if only because of how it made them look, not out of any real concern for their wayward son or who he was left in charge of.

I can imagine their sheer horror when one day, in the late 1960's, he arrived home on a motorcycle. He was my hero already but now he had become a god.

All I remember was that it was black, very noisy and smelled of burning oil, possibly an ancient BSA. He had a crash helmet with a metallic sunburst design and a denim waistcoat, that he had written 'Hell's Angels' on the back of with a black felt tip pen.

I don't think the bike worked very often, which was probably a good thing considering his track record involving moving objects.

Right in the middle of the whole mods versus rockers conflict, I had a brother on a motorbike and my sister on the back of a scooter.

I don't think he ever got into much trouble. Despite his size and the way he looked, he was just a gentle giant.

In 1983 he came to tell me that he was shortly to become my eldest sister. Perhaps he was expecting some sort of negative feedback, but I just hugged him tight and told him to do whatever made him happy and fuck the rest.

It was an incredibly brave thing to go through back then. He had to keep this news from our parents and the way in which they reacted after finding out has left me with a great deal of resentment towards them and a greater understanding of why he spent so little time at home.

Jim became Jo. One of the gentlest, generous and caring souls on this earth.

It took many years of self questioning and total ignorance before a chat with my sister revealed the real reasons why everyone flew the nest as soon as they could. None of it came as any great surprise. I was relieved that it wasn't just me that felt this way about my parents. I just wish somebody had told me earlier.

Another random memory of things I couldn't have seen (or maybe I did), was when riding my little red Triang scooter around the house. I lay it down on the floor to pick up a discarded piece of my sister's chewing gum, because it plainly needed chewing some more (This is how to build up your immune system.). I went to pick up my trusty red scooter only to find a large grey moth had taken a fancy to it and was sat on the handlebars. On closer inspection, the moth raised it's head to show the head of a demon, with huge sharp, canine teeth and glaring eyes. I ran indoors, in tears and refused to go anywhere near it for hours. Of course nobody believed me. For all I know it might have been a demon. You never know.

I've no doubt that stuff like this would have, more often than not, been a product of my fanciful imagination, but I seem to have more than my fair share of unusual and unexplainable happenings. I believe that the more of an open mind you have, the more open it is to new and unusual things. Everything in this universe has energy and you can either embrace it, or try to fight it. I would appear to attract weird energy by the megawatts. I like it that way.

Biker events attract weirdness and randomness by the bucket full. The reason for this is because they are one of the few places where you can just be yourself. Women can dress in clothes that would be frowned upon anywhere else and apart from that, the blokes seem to quite like it, for some strange reason?

Motorcycle custom shows produce some of the strangest and most brilliant creations to ever grace the tarmac. But it's the people that make the difference.

At a recent show in Portugal, you would have witnessed a guy dressed like a robot, on 6 foot stilts, walking around with a girl on a leash, who was randomly attacking passers by. A collection of scaffolding poles being pedalled around by 3 people, while a man played a piano on top of it and a guy riding a motorised television. Pretty much anything goes, within reason of course.

If it's the first time for somebody attending a rally, they might get the 'rally virgin' treatment. This can entail being made to spend all weekend wearing nothing but women's underwear, to various forms of public humiliation, usually involving copious amounts of alcohol plus getting very wet and dirty. A right of passage if you will.

Maybe not so much nowadays, but it was not unusual to find acts of a sexual nature taking place in full view of anyone who cared to watch. Rallys are very much 'family' events, so this doesn't happen as much anymore.

The latest event of randomness was on a visit to a bike show in Shropshire.

Opposite where we were all camping, there is a truck stop, which doubles as a convenience store and kebab house. Following a number of beers, the need for food took over, so we set off across the road to find sustenance.

There were a few trucks parked up for the weekend and sat in front of them were 4 drivers, who were beckoning us to come over. They were Eastern European truckers, 2 Romanians, 1 from Moldova and a fourth from Poland. They wanted us to share a drink with them and produced a small plastic bottle of clear liquid which was decanted into some paper cups. It was actually rather nice, in a rocket fuel sort of fashion. It was a little like swallowing a depth charge that exploded as it hit the stomach and sent an uncontrollable shudder through the whole nervous system. Of course we had another, it would have been rude not to.

After a few more cups of different coloured, suspicious looking liquids, we managed to get these guys into the show for free and the festivities continued. After all, we needed somebody to blame for the resulting hangovers, didn't we?

I honestly believe they thought we wouldn't be able to handle their homebrewed firewater. They obviously don't know British bikers very well. Certainly not my club brothers.

Of course it's not all fun and games. The biker lifestyle can bring with it a much darker side, depending on how you choose to live the life. A side most people will never get to see, because that's the way it works in our World. It can be a very private, insular and often dangerous place.

During my time on 2 wheels and involvement in the bike club scene, I have found myself in many situations where most people would run a mile, die of shock or hang up their helmets for good (some of them did).

I've been sat in a pub when a 4 foot section of a tree trunk was thrown through the window from the outside, showering everyone with shards of glass.

I have heard a man's skull crack open as he was beaten half to death with a knuckle duster.

I have sat in a car park, armed with various heavy tools, ready to kick a door down and rescue our brothers from trouble.

A lot of the time you just never know what might happen, but it's stuff like this that create the sort of bonds which never break.

There have been times when I've kissed my wife goodbye, not certain about my own chances of making it home, when there was more than a slight possibility of getting shot, stabbed or beaten.

One thing is for certain though, biker justice is swift and deadly. Threats are not just words, they're promises. It's difficult to explain this way of life to the uninitiated, but we call ourselves brothers for a reason and will defend each other without a thought for our own safety or consequence.

Now this might all sound like great fun and that a smashing time is had by all, but the reality of life with ADHD/ADD as a constant companion, is that there is always something waiting to reveal itself when you least expect it. There is a creature lurking in the wings. Just when you think everything is a good as it could possibly be, he will jump onto the stage and bite you in the bollocks.

In the guise of a huge, stinking, slobbering, black

dog, depression arrives from, seemingly nowhere and the dark side of the mind takes over. It drains the life from me, turns me into an antisocial misery. All I want to do is go to bed and shut out the World. It's nobody's fault but mine. Nothing has upset me or made me mad. I can think of nothing that has happened to make me feel so low. It just happens. Luckily this is quite a rare occurrence and after a few days of being a right grumpy and miserable old git, that doesn't want to talk to anyone or do anything, I get back to being that little ray of sunshine that we all know and love.... yeah, whatever.

It's as if my brain has reached saturation point and needs to shut down for a while. Sometimes your smartphone stops working properly and needs a restart. Too many tabs open. Too many apps running in the background. Too little memory left. Sounds about right. But enough about that. After all, it's depressing.

Despite my love of the motorcycle, my chosen form of transport, for my daily commute to work, is the bus. All things considered this should be my idea of hell, but it takes me just as long to get into my bike gear, uncover and unlock my machine, as it does to ride the 4 miles to my place of work.

My absolute hatred of crowds, noise and idiots in
general, is not exactly a good state of mind for
boarding public transport at rush hour. So I have
devised a number of coping mechanisms.

The first and easiest option is the use of an MP3
player, headphones, loud rock music and closed
eyes. This is my bus default mode and it works
well. Unless the battery runs out or I forget to take it
with me of course.

Then there's second method, which utilises the
creative, nonsensical and downright naughty side
of my rapidly changing thoughts. I create fictional
characters from the regular commuters. You never
know, this could be an exact description of who
they are in the real world. Which is rather scary.

For instance... There is this one guy, who I call
'Chuddy', due to his constant, rapid, open mouthed
mastication of chewing gum.
An average, middle aged bloke, who epitomizes the
word average in every possible way. With a pot
belly and, a quite comical, comb-over hairstyle,
black slip on shoes and Marks & Spencer slacks.
He tries to offset this look of greyness by wearing
an Isle of Man TT Races, or Las Vegas baseball
cap.

He will sit and play sudoku on his phone or read the
Daily Mail newspaper, only glancing upwards
whenever a young schoolgirl boards the bus.
In my mind, he is a bitter divorcee who has a
number of young girls locked in his basement. He
spends the weekend dressed in his ex wife's
clothes, whilst flogging himself with a leather whip.
He also likes to sit in McDonald's, nursing a cold
coffee at 1545, just as the school buses arrive.

Then there's Malcolm. If his name isn't Malcolm,
then it really should be.
With dirty ginger hair, gold rimmed spectacles,
protruding lips and no chin.
Malcolm gets kicked out of the house by his
snarling wife every morning.
She's a woman named Debbie, or Debs to her
friends. She has the same gold spectacles, but
sports a tight blonde ponytail and wears an
articulated clown necklace from Argos.
Malcolm tells all his workmates how he's the man
of the house, when in fact his wife kicks the shit out
of him every night. He has to cook, clean and fix
everything dressed in leather shorts, a gimp mask
and a snooker ball gag. His wife just watches reality
TV all day and night, drinking prosecco and using
Malcolm's spotty arse as a footstool.

He sleeps under the stairs in a dog bed and tells everyone he does karate, in a vain attempt to explain the bruising.

Mrs Angry is a regular passenger.
A hospital worker with a big square head and a man's haircut. Never smiling, she will stand at the front of the bus, even when there are plenty of seats, just to be a bloody nuisance.
I imagine her name is Sylvia and she has been forced to work into her 60's by her alcoholic and totally useless husband. I think she works in radiography and often subjects patients to x-ray overdoses, because she's too busy flicking through the pages of 'Take a Break' magazine whilst stuffing her face with chocolate hobnobs.
She has a dolphin tattoo on her shoulder for no reason whatsoever and goes on holiday to Benidorm twice a year with 'the girls'.
The only time she stops frowning at work is at the Christmas party, where she gets hammered on Jaeger bombs and thinks wearing a reindeer antler hair band and tinsel necklace makes her absolutely fucking hilarious.

Then there's 'Butcher'.
I only named him this because he permanently smells of raw meat.

Dressed in dirty clothes from charity shops, that are always at least 3 sizes too large. His eyes are constantly moving but never blink, in case he misses something.

He spends his day aimlessly wandering the streets and being asked to leave shops because of the smell.

He lives with his morbidly obese sister in a house full of cats, where the curtains are always closed.

He draws his own blood in order to feed his sisters habit and spends the night running naked through the village, hiding from unwary passers by and making small animal noises.

His hobbies include internet trolling, disecting frogs and making the lingerie pages of his sister's catalogue stick together. He never, ever, bathes.

'Blue Bike' …. He doesn't actually get on my bus but still manages to annoy the crap out of me.

Blue bike is a ruddy faced, middle aged cyclist that lies in wait for my bus. As he spots the bus heading towards him, he'll appear out of nowhere and pedal along, just in front of the bus, on roads that make it impossible for the driver to overtake him. If it becomes possible to get past him, it will be just before a bus stop with somebody waiting, leaving

just enough time for Blue Bike to ride past the bus
and get in front of it again.
He always looks like the effort is nearly killing him
and I imagine that he likes to wear black bin liners
under his stupid cycling gear, just because he likes
how it feels on his sweaty body.
If I was a bus diver, he'd be dead.

So there you have it. A small glimpse into the
workings of an ADHD fuelled imagination . No
really... you're welcome.

Back from the tangent and onto my lust for
motorcycles.
For whatever reason, I had this need to experience
a sportsbike.
I had ridden a few relatively fast machines, but
nothing quite prepared me for the Kawasaki ZX9r.
 A 900cc rocket ship with a fast revving engine and
race honed rolling chassis created for just one
purpose. Going fast.
The first time I twisted the throttle, after clicking up
to second gear, was unlike anything I had
experienced before. Like a scalded cat on
amphetamines gets barely close. Not only that, it
handled like a dream and remains the only bike on
which I have, almost, had my knee down on the
tarmac. Made all the more impressive by the fact

that it was going around a roundabout and I am usually rather timid when it comes to right hand turns, due entirely to my right shoulder injury.

The only problem with this style of bike is the discomfort. Most of your weight is transferred onto the arms and wrists, plus there's the neck ache to contend with. You will often see sportsbike riders, when riding slowly, with one arm on their hips. This is not an attempt to look camp, but a rest for tired wrists, arms and neck.

With the all too frequent aches and pains, the question arises as to why people bother. Simple... it's the speed. It's like a drug and nothing else can replace it. Not so much the top speed but the insane acceleration which leaves every spotty teenager, in their Vauxhall Corsas, with body kits and drainpipe exhausts, wondering why they even bothered revving their inadequate little engine next to you at the traffic lights.

The major downside to owning a bike with so many adrenaline creation opportunities, is the ever increasing possibility of losing your licence. There is also the sensation, following a good blast of 120mph or more (so a friend tells me of course), that 70mph suddenly feels like you could just step off the bike and walk, which is not at all advisable. Finding yourself on a slip road coming off the dual carriageway, still doing 100mph is not uncommon and 100 mph plus happens in a matter of seconds. More good reasons why I don't ride them anymore. I have owned three ZX9rs in total, which says a lot about how much I admire them. All mark 1 versions by the way. The only thing I have ridden to match them was a Mark 1 Honda Fireblade, but it's a Honda and we've already covered that.

It always amuses me to see sportsbike riding 'power rangers' with digital video cameras attached to their helmets, speeding along busy country roads and taking stupid risks to show off to their mates. What better way for the nice Mr Policeman to gather evidence of what a complete and utter tool you've been, after pulling you over for riding like a twat. Your new bike and 600 quid leathers will soon be gracing the pages of eBay while you're examining bus timetables and scrolling through job sites. Silly boys.

Bikers of my era eventually succumb to the ravages of ageing, injuries past and the effects of riding in all weathers over our lifetimes. Not to mention all the bad things we have put our bodies through over the years. Luckily there is a new generation of cruiser style motorcycles that can still provide us with some grin forming performance, whilst retaining some degree of comfort and a large helping of cool.

To be honest, I still feel like a 19 year old when I go out on my Yamaha Warrior. The 1.7 litres of V twin engine provides enough torque to drag a smile out of the hardest grimace and most importantly, it still scares the shit out of me at times.

And that my friend is what it's all about.

CHAPTER 11

'It's like in martial arts. You learn to implement techniques you learn under stress. If you can't do them under stress, you haven't learned anything. And that's where the writing comes in. Can you do this amongst the noise? Can you tune in and find out who you are as a writer.'
Maynard James Keenan (singer/songwriter).

...and that sums it up perfectly. You have to learn to live with the noise.

Certain kinds of noise are a comfort to me and create a balancing effect inside the mind.

I sleep better with white noise, be that an electric fan or actual white noise through headphones.

Then there are binaural sounds, which can have some very interesting and unusual effects. Most natural sounds are good, it's only the man made stuff that bothers me and there's always plenty of that to choose from.

But now it gets weird. There are certain sounds that send me into an almost trance like state, they don't make sense to me or anyone else but it happens.

One particular sound is the noise of somebody eating a bag of crisps or something similar. There is something about the noise the packaging makes that relaxes me. Figure that one out ?

Another is the sound of somebody breathing, if they have a bit of trouble doing so, a bit like an English Bulldog for instance. There are a few more things but none that get to me like these.

The only plausible reason for the packet thing , that I can possibly imagine, is that when I was a little kid, my Grandmother used to live with my parents and always spent time with me, playing cards or whatever else we used to pass the time with. She was a particularly heavy smoker and got through quite a few packets of Woodbines, unfiltered, lung destroying cigarettes during the day. Maybe the sound of her unwrapping the packets has created a link between that feeling of comfort and happiness that was so alien to me, compared to being with my mother and father.

I like my music loud, it brings me peace. If you can't 'feel' it, it ain't loud enough. This is why I like to be the DJ in our clubhouse, or at events. Playing my favourite tracks through extra large speakers is most satisfying, especially if others are enjoying it too.

Despite my lack of self confidence and introvert nature, I have this dream of singing on stage with my own rock band. I have no problem getting up on stage, believe it or not. It's like an out of body experience, as if I'm watching another 'me' up there, that has stepped out of the shy, quiet cocoon and forgot about everything that ever held him back.

That energy reaches me from somewhere I can't quite understand, but I'm grateful for it regardless. We did try starting our own band, made up entirely of club members, but couldn't find a guitarist. It might happen one day. I sincerely hope so.

Armed with the recent discovery of my condition, I can look back on my life and start to make sense of it. I'm not making excuses for things, just trying to figure out the reasons why they happened.

In hindsight, I must have appeared to be a very selfish, self centred dick head.

I was always doing stuff without thinking about how it would impact on others. I was so wrapped up in my own thoughts, that everything else got blocked out.

I must admit that, occasionally, this still happens. I try not to fall into this mental trap, but sometimes my mind gets the better of me. All I can do is apologise in advance and assure you that I didn't mean to be like that.

Buddhist teachings say that we should question everything. Believe me, I do. Mostly myself.
After more than half a century of getting things wrong, lacking understanding, and generally fucking things up, I expect the worse to happen every time. It comes as more of a surprise to me if it doesn't.
I never expect to win, succeed or excel in anything anymore. This is not me being a depressing loser. It's programmed into my brain.
I don't see it as a bad thing. After all, expectation is the mother of disappointment.

The only thing I ever succeeded at, where so many have failed, is the Royal Air Force aircrew selection test. Not only did I pass the test to become a navigator, I did so at the tender age of 16.
I passed the bare minimum of GCE 'O' levels that were needed to apply and made my way to Biggin Hill, in Kent. I imagine most parents would have taken their young son to such an important and life changing event. Not mine.
I had to get various trains, negotiate the London Underground and catch a number of buses to get there. It took forever, not helped by it being the middle of winter and dark by 4pm.

On arrival, late in the evening, I was shown to my accommodation and came face to face with beings from a completely different dimension.

I kid you not. The first person I spoke to had the name Farquar Farquraharson.

There I was, a normal lad, from a working class family, with a secondary school education, being quizzed by a privately schooled, highly educated and privileged, posh kid. He wanted to know which school I attended and what business my father was involved in.

I don't think Christleton High School and cleaning the inside of petrol refinery production tanks, was the answer he was expecting.

During the evening, the room gradually filled up with Farquar clones. I sat quietly on my own, looking on in disbelief at these chinless, chattering aliens.

Nevertheless, I breezed through all the tests with ease. I was still far too young to start training, so got told by the training officers to join up as soon as I could, then get back to them when I was over 18.

The most satisfying thing about the whole weekend was not so much that I passed with flying colours. It was because Farquar didn't.

I don't actually think I've ever really failed at
anything I really wanted to do.
I failed a couple of exams, but only in subjects that
held no interest for me.
It all depends on what you regard as failure. To me,
you only fail at something if you don't try at all. As
long as you've done the best you can, that's all that
matters.
I simply cannot abide those over confident,
ambitious types, that will do anything to get what
they want. Including using others.
Manipulating, lying and cheating their way up the
ladder. Trampling on everyone around them without
a thought for their fellow man.
I have no problem with people trying to better
themselves, just the way some of them go about it.
If there is one thing I learnt, while employed at the
Royal Mail, is that ability is no guarantee of
success.
After many years of experience, training new
starters and gaining a widespread knowledge of the
postal service, I decided to try my hand at junior
management.
This involved completing a written test, followed by
an interview.
A few days after the interview, I was called into my
line manager's office and told to take a seat.

He asked me how I thought the test and interview went. I said that I found the test remarkably easy and the interview seemed to go OK.

With a small hint of disbelief, he went on to tell me that I had scored higher than anyone ever had in the written test and was successful at the interview stage.

Approximately a week later, I received a letter telling me that, unfortunately I had been unsuccessful in my application for a management role. Please apply again for any future positions.

What I learned from this experience is that it takes a lot more than being good at something to get what you want. At least it did in that sector.

I began to realise that the people in charge of such decisions, were all very similar people. Very ambitious and clever people.

From their perspective, anyone that could do so well in the application exam was seen as a threat to their future success. It was someone else to get in their way for future promotions.

It became crystal clear to me what was going on, when a colleague of mine, who confided in me that he simply couldn't answer the test questions, got the job instead of me. Even he couldn't believe it. Lower management started filling up with incompetent idiots, that had no idea how to manage

staff, talk to people or act professionally. Basically,
they posed no threat to those above them.
The only way anyone of them could expect to climb
up the ladder, was to become a sycophantic, yes
man, that started playing golf with higher
management.
I know, this sounds like sour grapes. In reality I
wasn't that bothered. I have never been that
ambitious or competitive. In all honesty, I just
fancied doing something different. They had
nothing to worry about.
I've never liked golf anyway.

Today I measure success in how I feel and, more
importantly, how I make others feel.
I feel no need to put myself under a load of
pressure and work ridiculous hours, just to earn a
bit more money. My time is much more important.
My free time and time spent with the woman I love.
I don't see the point of working yourself to death,
when death itself can take it all away from you in an
instant.
I used to see postal workers, working 6, twelve
hour night shifts, up until the day they retired.
Desperately trying to get a decent pension sum,

only to die a couple of months later. It had all been for nothing.

This society we live in provides us with a very fragile existence.
In my line of work, I often see working people, with comfortable lifestyles, reduced to having nothing and living on the streets, within months of losing their job. It's frightening how quickly it can happen.
All we can really do is embrace the moment and be content with what we have.
Flashy new cars, the latest smartphone, and a 52 inch, 4k HD Television are all very nice things to have, but do they really matter?
Happiness to me, is love, friendship and good health.
After years of swapping motorcycles, I have eventually found the one I'm totally happily with (nobody believes me but it's true). I'm married to a strong, independent and incredibly sexy woman.
We have a warm roof over our heads and food in the fridge.
Life is good.

Dale Carnegie, a famous American writer and
lecturer, once wrote,
"It isn't what you have, or who you are, or where
you are, or what you are doing that makes you
happy or unhappy. It is what you think about."

I think a lot. Maybe a little too much.

EPILOGUE

'I'm sorry…I wasn't paying attention to what I was thinking.'
— **Shelley Curtiss.**

Today I have good life, not extravagant but with everything I need.

My way of life might seem alien to some, but not to the people who matter to me.

When you're in the company of kindred souls, the outside world ceases to matter and there is no other feeling quite like it.

It was summed up recently by my club brother Tony. He said, "How do you tell people what it's like..? How do you explain the love ?"

Unless you're part of it and fully embrace it, you simply cannot.

I could try and give you a shit load of advice about how to cope with ADD/ADHD, but I believe the way it affects people is a very personal thing.

Where I work, I often come across youngsters who claim to have ADHD, but I know otherwise. Most of the time they are just arrogant little pricks with no respect for anything or anybody, looking for a way to excuse and justify their disrespectful behaviour. If it was a simple condition, there would be a simple, single medication to treat it. The reality is that there are a number of treatments, which can only be judged by trial and error. Some of the side effects are terrible and can make things a lot worse.

The only thing I have found that helps to calm my brain activity, to some degree, is CBD oil (cannabidiol). This is taken from the cannabis plant but has the active ingredient THC removed (the part that gets you stoned). It works for me but might not work for you.

The only real advice I can offer, is to just roll with it. Use it to your advantage and talk about it, openly and without embarrassment. What's the worst that can happen?

Speaking about a problem out loud, takes away most of its power. Demons like to lurk in quiet, dark places, so make them feel exposed. They hate it.

Yes, I'm still impulsive, get agitated when there is nothing for me to do, daydream a lot and sometimes appear not to be listening, but I'm trying